AF515220

Reducing Mortality in Acute Kidney Injury

Giovanni Landoni • Antonio Pisano
Alberto Zangrillo • Rinaldo Bellomo
Editors

Reducing Mortality in Acute Kidney Injury

Springer

Editors
Giovanni Landoni
Dept of Anesthesia & Intensive care
IRCCS San Raffaele Scientific Institute
Milano
Italy

Alberto Zangrillo
Dept of Anesthesia & Intensive care
IRCCS San Raffaele Scientific Institute
Milano
Italy

Antonio Pisano
Cardiac Anesthesia & ICU
AORN Dei Colli, Monaldi Hospital
Naples
Italy

Rinaldo Bellomo
Austin Hospital
Heidelberg
Victoria
Australia

ISBN 978-3-319-33427-1 ISBN 978-3-319-33429-5 (eBook)
DOI 10.1007/978-3-319-33429-5

Library of Congress Control Number: 2016946426

© Springer International Publishing Switzerland 2016
This work is subject to copyright. All rights are reserved by the Publisher, whether the whole or part of the material is concerned, specifically the rights of translation, reprinting, reuse of illustrations, recitation, broadcasting, reproduction on microfilms or in any other physical way, and transmission or information storage and retrieval, electronic adaptation, computer software, or by similar or dissimilar methodology now known or hereafter developed.
The use of general descriptive names, registered names, trademarks, service marks, etc. in this publication does not imply, even in the absence of a specific statement, that such names are exempt from the relevant protective laws and regulations and therefore free for general use.
The publisher, the authors and the editors are safe to assume that the advice and information in this book are believed to be true and accurate at the date of publication. Neither the publisher nor the authors or the editors give a warranty, express or implied, with respect to the material contained herein or for any errors or omissions that may have been made.

Printed on acid-free paper

This Springer imprint is published by Springer Nature
The registered company is Springer International Publishing AG Switzerland

Preface

Acute kidney injury (AKI) carries a heavy burden of morbidity and mortality in any clinical setting. In particular, AKI represents a big deal for surgeons, anesthesiologists, and intensivists worldwide, since it may occur in more than a third of patients undergoing major surgery and in up to two thirds of intensive care unit (ICU) patients, especially those with sepsis. Furthermore, AKI is relatively common in many other clinical situations including liver disease, hematologic malignancies, and exposure to contrast media. Accordingly, other specialists such as gastroenterologists, hematologists, radiologists, and interventional cardiologists have to take care of AKI in their daily clinical practice.

AKI reduces patients' quality of life, increases hospital length of stay and care costs, it may progress towards chronic kidney disease and, above all, it increases both short- and long-term mortality. In patients undergoing major surgery, for example, AKI is associated with an almost fourfold increase in 90-day mortality, while mortality rate is more than doubled in ICU patients with any stage of AKI and it may reach 60% in those requiring renal replacement therapy (RRT).

Unfortunately, so far very few interventions have been clearly proven to be effective in preventing either AKI or its progression towards the need for RRT or end-stage renal failure requiring "chronic" hemodialysis. A review of the best-quality and widely agreed evidence about the therapeutic interventions (drugs, techniques, and strategies) that may affect mortality in patients with or at risk for AKI was recently achieved using an innovative, web-based consensus process. This "democracy-based" approach has been already applied to the identification of all interventions which may influence mortality in other clinical settings such as the perioperative period of any adult surgery and critical care.

Like "*Reducing Mortality in the Perioperative Period*" and "*Reducing Mortality in Critically Ill Patients,*" this third book explores in detail all the identified interventions which could be implemented (or avoided) in order to reduce mortality in patients with or at risk for AKI. The covered topics range from all aspects of renal replacement therapy (modality, intensity, timing, anticoagulation) to drugs or strategies which have proven to be effective in preventing or treating AKI in various clinical settings (cirrhosis, sepsis, multiple myeloma, angiography, surgery, burns) to those therapeutic approaches (loop diuretics, hydroxyethyl starches, fluid overload) which could cause or aggravate AKI. Every chapter deals with an individual drug, technique, or strategy and it is structured in: background knowledge, main evidence from literature, and a practical how-to-do section. We also briefly describe the innovative consensus process that gave strength to our systematic review.

We thank all the hundreds of colleagues from all over the world who spent their time to help us in this consensus building process and the prestigious international authors who wrote the 22 chapters of this book. We hope that it may represent a significant contribution to spread the awareness of acute kidney injury as a major medical issue, to help clinicians in making therapeutic choices which may hopefully improve survival of their patients and, finally, to give useful hints for future research.

Milan, Italy Giovanni Landoni
Naples, Italy Antonio Pisano
Milan, Italy Alberto Zangrillo
Heidelberg, Australia Rinaldo Bellomo

Contents

Part IV Update

Part I

Introduction

Acute Kidney Injury: The Plague of the New Millennium

1

Zaccaria Ricci and Claudio Ronco

1.1 The "Atra Mors"

Although not infectious, acute kidney injury (AKI) is pandemic. Interestingly, like infection by *Yersinia pestis*, AKI has "spread" to both high- and low-income countries (even if likely secondary to significantly different pathogenetic pathways), and its outcomes are bad worldwide [1]: the deadly burden of AKI affects up to 5,000 cases per million people per year and kills up to 50% of patients requiring renal replacement therapy (RRT) secondary to AKI [2]. Again, similarly to the Black Death (*Atra Mors*, in Latin) pandemics which broke out between the fourteenth and the nineteenth century, we are fighting against a barely known enemy without a specific therapy to administer. Very differently from the plague, AKI is a syndrome and is caused by multiple etiologies, frequently occurring simultaneously. However, the exact damage occurring to kidneys' structure and function, through multiple and complex pathophysiologic mechanisms, is largely unknown. This uncertainty led the medical community (only recently, about 10 years ago) to search for a standard AKI definition [3] which is able to conventionally describe that the abrupt decrease of kidney function is not an "on-off" disease, but it has a spectrum of phenotypes (currently known as "AKI stages"; see Chap. 2). The standard definition is unable to identify and differentiate AKI etiologies and somehow causes a "one-fits-all" issue: detractors of "consensus-based" definitions

Z. Ricci, MD (✉)
Department of Cardiology, Cardiac Surgery, and Pediatric Cardiac Intensive Care Unit, Bambino Gesù Children's Hospital, IRCCS, Piazza S.Onofrio 4, Rome 00165, Italy
e-mail: zaccaria.ricci@opbg.net

C. Ronco, MD
Department of Nephrology, Dialysis and Transplantation, San Bortolo Hospital, Viale Ferdinando Rodolfi, 37, Vicenza 36100, Italy

International Renal Research Institute, San Bortolo Hospital, Viale Ferdinando Rodolfi, 37, Vicenza 36100, Italy
e-mail: cronco@goldnet.it

© Springer International Publishing Switzerland 2016

G. Landoni et al. (eds.), *Reducing Mortality in Acute Kidney Injury*,
DOI 10.1007/978-3-319-33429-5_1

argue that, for example, a stage II septic AKI might not be clinically comparable to a stage II postabdominal surgery AKI [3]. At least, however, some light has been shed on the obscure epidemiology of AKI, and it is now clear that AKI occurs with a different incidence in different clinical settings [4], inevitably leading, regardless of etiology, to significantly worse outcomes as compared to non-affected (plagued) patients. Exactly as it happened before the availability of antibiotics during plague pandemics, prevention of AKI might represent today the most significant way to improve outcomes in those populations at risk of developing an acute renal dysfunction.

1.2 Why AKI Kills

From the milestone paper by Meitnitz, back in 2002 [5], clinicians understood two fundamental concepts: (1) if two critically ill patients with the same severity of disease (assessed through common metrics such as APACHE score) are admitted to the same intensive care unit (ICU), the one with AKI has an independently higher risk of dying: the "only" fact the kidneys are not working, regardless how good is medical treatment in your ward, how early, intense, and optimal is your RRT, and how appropriate is your antibiotic therapy, your patient has AKI and, as such, his chances of surviving decrease; (2) this frustrating scenario (again similar to that of Indian fellows staring powerlessly at hundreds of patients suffering from *Yersinia*'s lesions) taught us that the commonly used "severity scores" have overlooked for years the actual impact of renal function on patient outcomes: a novel and specific AKI risk stratification was absolutely needed [3]. Interestingly, the impact of isolated AKI (e.g., in case of glomerulonephritis in a previously healthy patient) on patients' outcome is significantly different compared to AKI occurring in patients with multiple comorbidities (e.g., cardiorenal or hepatorenal syndrome) or multiple organ failure (MOF). As a matter of fact, it is currently unknown if this harmful disease affects critically ill patients in association with the most severe clinical pictures, already hampered by a worst outcome, or is itself the cause of increased death rate. It is possible that the truth is in the middle: kidneys are victims and culprits in the course of MOF, being most frequently injured by systemic diseases (e.g., sepsis) and causing themselves, in a sort of vicious circle, damage to other organs. AKI is a "pan-metabolic, pan-endocrine, and pan-organ" problem [6]. Vaara and coauthors [7] elegantly described the "population-attributable mortality" of AKI by attempting to compare AKI and non-AKI patients through a most complex system of propensity matching in a large database from several Finnish ICUs that included more than 60 variables. These authors concluded that almost 20 % of mortality in the ICU population is caused by AKI. In particular, AKI seems to affect and enhance inflammatory processes and to cause a profound depression of immunocompetence. This is associated with the release of cytokines and inflammatory mediators, increase in oxidative stress, activation of white line cells, neutrophil extravasation, generalized endothelial injury, increased vascular permeability, and tissue edema formation [8]. The alteration of the delicate equilibrium in multiple immuno-homeostatic mechanisms further justifies the role of "injured" kidneys as "activators" of MOF: the lungs, heart, liver, and brain are all equally exposed to this largely unexplored syndrome [9].

The alteration of fluid management is another key issue in patients suffering from AKI [10]: critically ill patients are necessarily administered with large amounts of fluids (fluid challenges, transfusions, antibiotics, parenteral nutrition, vasoactive drugs, etc.). Fluid overload (the percentage of cumulative fluid balance over patients' body weight) may result from overzealous fluid administration or oliguria or a combination of the two (see Chap. 19). It has been speculated that these two aspects may combine, again, into a vicious circle: it is possible that the largest fluid replacement is needed in most severe patients who are those at highest risk for AKI. Furthermore, infused fluids for volume replacement have been recently claimed to be in cause, per se, for nephrotoxicity and renal damage [11, 12]. Third, fluid overload and AKI share endothelial dysfunction due to inflammation or ischemia/reperfusion with glycocalyx alteration and subsequent capillary leakage [13]. As a matter of fact, organ edema (affecting the lungs, heart, liver, brain, and kidneys themselves) impairs organ function, and it is considered a fundamental constituent of MOF. It is actually difficult to understand who comes first (AKI or fluid overload) but it is clear that in case of severe AKI, the only way to manage fluid balance is aggressive ultrafiltration through RRT [14].

1.3 The Mark of AKI

Differently from plague infection, patients who survive AKI carry the signs of the disease in the following years. Recently, Heung and coworkers on behalf of the Centers for Disease Control and Prevention CKD Surveillance Team [15] showed that, in a cohort of about 100,000 hospitalized patients, the majority (70.8 %) had fast recovery (within 2 days), 12.2 % had intermediate recovery (3–10 days), 11.0 % had slow or no recovery (above 10 days), and the remaining 6.0 % were lost to follow-up: one patient over ten (maybe more) does not recover an intra-hospital AKI episode and is destined to chronic kidney disease (CKD) thereafter. Impressively, the authors remarked that, at 1-year follow-up, the presence of any AKI episode was strongly associated with the development of CKD, with a relative risk of 1.43 (95 % confidence interval [CI] 1.39–1.48), 2.00 (95 % CI 1.88–2.12), and 2.65 (95 % CI 2.51–2.80) for fast, intermediate, and slow recovery, respectively. Thus, even a transient AKI episode, lasting less than 2 days, leaves a scar in patients' kidneys that subsequently increases the risk of further renal damage. Follow-up should be warranted to all AKI patients.

1.4 How to Reduce AKI Mortality

Dr. Alexandre Yersin, from the Pasteur Institute, significantly contributed to plague therapy by isolating the bacterium in 1894 and was thereafter honored by giving his name to the etiologic agent. Today, the therapeutic solution of AKI is far from being identified, and we possibly will never see a single name on such treatment. However, several approaches can be currently suggested.

Primum non nocere: the avoidance of useless and not effective treatments may certainly help clinicians to focus on more consistent approaches [16].

In the same light, the earliest diagnosis of AKI is currently considered a fundamental aspect of plague's management: the identification of renal dysfunction from its milder forms [17] or, better, before the manifest sings are apparent [18] is useful in order to promote preventive measures (e.g., administer antibiotics targeting serum levels, reduce contrast media, avoid starches administration, etc.) and to keep clinicians aware about kidney's health in the eventual attempt of precluding the worsening of AKI severity. Great expectations are currently trusted on renal biomarkers for early detection of AKI (see Chap. 2) [19] and "acute kidney stress" [20].

Third, act upon disease pathogenesis. Sepsis, fluid overload, surgery, cardiac dysfunction, and trauma: they all have partially different clinical pictures and deserve tailored attention. Possibly, a surgical patient will benefit from an accurate and aggressive goal-directed fluid replacement (see Chap. 10), whereas a septic one should be "fluid restricted," mostly avoiding starch infusion (see Chaps. 19 and 20). Research is ongoing in every single setting, and scientific updating is certainly an important part of clinicians' efforts: we should attempt to administer the most appropriate therapy according to the most recent evidences.

Then, do not delay RRT (see Chap. 5) and treat fluid accumulation. Importantly, RRT dose should be closely monitored during the entire ICU stay and changed basing on clinical needs (see Chap. 6) [21].

Finally, read this book carefully: the most updated therapeutic approaches are described in the next chapters in order to increase clinician's awareness and good clinical practice against AKI, the plague of critically ill patients.

References

1. Lameire NH, Bagga A, Cruz D et al (2013) Acute kidney injury: an increasing global concern. Lancet 382:170–179
2. Bellomo R, Kellum JA, Ronco C (2012) Acute kidney injury. Lancet 380:756–766
3. Cruz DN, Ricci Z, Ronco C (2009) Clinical review: RIFLE and AKIN – time for reappraisal. Crit Care 13:211
4. Hoste EA, Bagshaw SM, Bellomo R et al (2015) Epidemiology of acute kidney injury in critically ill patients: the multinational AKI-EPI study. Intensive Care Med 41:1411–1423
5. Metnitz PGH, Krenn CG, Steltzer H et al (2002) Effect of acute renal failure requiring renal replacement therapy on outcome in critically ill patients. Crit Care Med 30:2051–2058
6. Druml W, Lenz K, Laggner AN (2015) Our paper 20 years later: from acute renal failure to acute kidney injury—the metamorphosis of a syndrome. Intensive Care Med 41(11):1941–1949
7. Vaara ST, Kaukonen K, Bendel S et al (2014) The attributable mortality of acute kidney injury: a sequentially matched analysis. Crit Care Med 42:1–8
8. Druml W (2014) Systemic consequences of acute kidney injury. Curr Opin Crit Care 20:613–619

9. Feltes CM, Van Eyk J, Rabb H (2008) Distant-organ changes after acute kidney injury. Nephron Physiol 109(4):p80–p84
10. Ostermann M, Straaten HMO, Forni LG (2015) Fluid overload and acute kidney injury: cause or consequence? Crit Care 19:443
11. Young P, Bailey M, Beasley R et al (2015) Effect of a buffered crystalloid solution vs saline on acute kidney injury among patients in the intensive care unit. JAMA 314(16):1701–1710
12. Myburgh JA, Mythen MG (2013) Resuscitation fluids. N Engl J Med 369:1243–1251
13. Ricci Z, Romagnoli S, Ronco C (2012) Perioperative intravascular volume replacement and kidney insufficiency. Best Pract Res Clin Anaesthesiol 26:463–474
14. RENAL replacement therapy study Investigators (2012) An observational study fluid balance and patient outcomes in the randomized evaluation of normal vs. augmented level of replacement therapy trial. Crit Care Med 40:1753–1760
15. Heung M, Steffick DE, Zivin K et al (2016) Acute kidney injury recovery pattern and subsequent risk of CKD: an analysis of veterans health administration data. Am J Kidney Dis 67:742–752
16. Landoni G, Bove T, Székely A et al (2013) Reducing mortality in acute kidney injury patients: systematic review and international web-based survey. J Cardiothorac Vasc Anesth 27:1384–1398
17. Kellum JA, Lameire N, Aspelin P et al (2012) KDIGO clinical practice guideline for acute kidney injury. Kidney Int Suppl 2:1–138
18. Chawla LS, Goldstein SL, Kellum JA, Ronco C (2015) Renal angina: concept and development of pretest probability assessment in acute kidney injury. Crit Care 19:93
19. Kellum JA (2015) Diagnostic criteria for acute kidney injury: present and future. Crit Care Clin 31:621–632
20. Katz N, Ronco C (2015) Acute kidney stress—a useful term based on evolution in the understanding of acute kidney injury. Crit Care 20:23
21. Villa G, Ricci Z, Ronco C (2015) Renal replacement therapy. Crit Care Clin 31:839–848

Acute Kidney Injury: Definitions, Incidence, Diagnosis, and Outcome

2

Francis X. Dillon and Enrico M. Camporesi

2.1 Introduction

Surgeons, anesthesiologists, intensivists, radiologists, interventional cardiologists, and nephrologists, among others, are keenly interested in preserving renal function in patients undergoing surgical interventions or other procedures, as well as in intensive care unit (ICU) patients. The well-known strong association between acute kidney injury (AKI) and its sequel, chronic kidney disease (CKD) with mortality and with severe cardiac and other organ morbidity [1–5] makes practitioners even more mindful of kidney function in these patients. No effective new therapy for AKI has been introduced so far; thus better avenues for progress may be novel diagnostic tests and a clearer understanding of the factors associated with the development of AKI in both surgical and critically ill patients and how to prevent it.

Around 2000, the lack of novel pharmacologic strategies for AKI therapy seemed to awaken a critical mass of epidemiologists and nephrologists: worldwide a reassessment of the most fundamental questions about AKI was spurred, and nephrology literature from 2004 onward was eventually unfolded.

F.X. Dillon, MD (✉)
TEAMHealth Inc./Florida Gulf-to-Bay Anesthesia Associates LLC, Tampa General Hospital, 1 Tampa General Circle, Suite A327, Tampa, FL 33606, USA

Department of Surgery, University of South Florida, Tampa, FL 33606, USA
e-mail: fxdillon@gmail.com

E.M. Camporesi, MD
TEAMHealth Inc./Florida Gulf-to-Bay Anesthesia Associates LLC, Tampa General Hospital, 1 Tampa General Circle, Suite A327, Tampa, FL 33606, USA

Department of Surgery, University of South Florida, Tampa, FL 33606, USA

Department of Anesthesiology, Molecular Pharmacology and Physiology, University of South Florida, Tampa, FL 33606, USA
e-mail: ecampore@health.usf.edu

© Springer International Publishing Switzerland 2016

G. Landoni et al. (eds.), *Reducing Mortality in Acute Kidney Injury*,
DOI 10.1007/978-3-319-33429-5_2

The first most urgent questions were related on AKI definition, how best AKI could be classified, what is its etiology, and how best to prevent it. If indeed prevention is the only way of reducing the burden of AKI and of its sequelae (outside of renal replacement therapy [RRT]), then clarifying definition was the obligatory first step.

2.2 The Evolution of AKI Definition

The lack of uniformity in naming and defining AKI has been a serious impediment to progress in the field's epidemiology [6]. From the standpoint of nomenclature, the older term "acute renal failure" (ARF) was predominant until 2005 when the term AKI emerged. The term ARF is now obsolete as an acronym in medicine and nephrology.

The significance of this change in nomenclature was felt by many in the nephrology community to be of great, even revolutionary importance because generally the older references in the nephrology and critical care literature had often defined ARF less precisely than the newer term AKI would be defined. For example, in a 1999 review Nissenson defined ARF in the critical care setting as "the abrupt decline in glomerular filtration rate (GFR) resulting from ischemic or toxic injury to the kidney" [7]. Some authors defined ARF as azotemia with or without oliguria. Other authors had recorded increases in blood urea nitrogen (BUN) to diagnose ARF and omitted serum creatinine (sCr) measurements. In others, the timing of sCr or BUN samples was incompletely documented. Some authors noted rehydration as a precondition for diagnosing ARF, while others did not specify the presence or absence of rehydration as a part of this definition. In the seminal critical care paper in which the first exact definition of AKI was introduced, Bellomo et al. [8] noted that some 30 definitions of ARF had hitherto been used at different times in the literature.

From 2002 onward, three different consensus definitions, from three different workgroups, have emerged and become accepted, and the reader needs to be aware of the differences between them when comparing studies. No single consensus definition has yet emerged as the standard definition, but the use of KDIGO definition [9] (see below) is currently recommended for epidemiologic and research purposes.

2.2.1 The ADQI Workgroup Was Formed to Address a Lack of Consensus Over How Best to Treat AKI with RRT: Eventually, the Group Produced RIFLE, an Acronym Defining AKI by Its Severity in Stages

The Acute Dialysis Quality Initiative (ADQI) [8, 10] Workgroup was founded in 2000 by representatives from the US National Institutes of Health (NIH), American Society of Nephrology (ASN), and the Society of Critical Care Medicine (SCCM), among others. In 2004, its founding members identified a definition and classification system for AKI. It employed the mnemonic acronym RIFLE (for "risk," "injury," "failure," "loss" of renal function, and "end-stage" kidney disease). The various levels of AKI were defined according to azotemia (serum creatinine) *and* urinary output (UO) criteria (Table 2.1) [8]. Note that the most severe criteria in either the azotemia or oliguria columns should be applied when assigning a RIFLE stratum: i.e., one should use whichever criterion that assigns the most severe class of AKI.

2.2.2 The AKIN Diagnostic and Staging Criteria for AKI Emphasize Azotemia

The members of the Acute Kidney Injury Network (AKIN) first met in 2005 and proposed a diagnostic criterion for AKI [11] (see Table 2.2) in order to improve some of RIFLE drawbacks. The AKIN workgroup classified AKI into three degrees of severity called stages 1, 2, and 3 (Table 2.3). Note that, as the AQDI definition did, these resemble the "R," "I," and "F" strata, which also take into account creatinine increase over baseline as well as oliguria. The AKIN guideline also stipulates adequate fluid resuscitation prior to diagnosis of AKI.

Table 2.1 The acute dialysis quality initiative (ADQI) workgroup criteria and classification for AKI

RIFLE criterion[a]	GFR criterion	Urine output criterion	Sensitivity or specificity
Risk	Increased sCr × 1.5 or GFR decrease ≥25 %	UO <0.5 mL/kg h × 6 h	High sensitivity
Injury	Increased sCr × 2 or GFR decrease ≥50 %	UO <0.5 mL/kg h × 12 h	
Failure	Increased sCr × 3 or GFR decrease ≥75 % or sCr ≥4 mg/dL (acute rise of ≥0.5 mg/dL)	UO <0.3 mL/kg h × 24 h or anuria × 12 h	High specificity
Loss	Persistent ARF: complete loss of renal function >4 weeks		
End-stage	End-stage kidney disease		

Modified from Bellomo et al. [8]

GFR glomerular filtration rate, *UO* urine output, *sCr* serum creatinine, and *ARF* acute renal failure

[a]Select the highest (worst) RIFLE level using either the GFR or urine output criteria

Table 2.2 AKIN diagnostic criteria for AKI

An abrupt (within 48 h) reduction in kidney function defined as (one of the three below):
An absolute increase in serum creatinine of 0.3 mg/dl (26.4 μmol/l) *or*
A percentage increase in serum creatinine of 50 % (1.5-fold from baseline) *or*
A reduction in urine output (documented oliguria of <0.5 mL/kg h for >6 h)
Criteria to be applied in the context of the clinical presentation and following adequate fluid resuscitation

Modified from Molitoris et al. [11] and Mehta et al. [72]

Table 2.3 Staging of AKI according to AKIN

Stage	sCr criteria	Urine output criteria
1	A serum Cr increase of 0.3 mg/dl (26.4 μmol/L) *or* An increase of sCr 150–200 % from baseline	UO <0.5 mL/kg per hour for >6 h
2	A sCr increase of 200 % over baseline	UO <0.5 mL/kg per hour for >12 h
3	A sCr increase of 300 % over baseline *or* A sCr ≥4.0 mg/dL (354 μmol/L) with an acute increase ≥0.5 mg/dL (44 μmol/L) *or* A need for RRT	UO <0.3 mL/kg per hour for 24 h or anuria for 12 h

Modified from Mehta et al. [72]
sCr serum creatinine, *UO* urine output, and *RRT* renal replacement therapy

Table 2.4 Diagnosis and staging of AKI according to the KDIGO workgroup

The diagnosis of AKI is made by any one of the following:		
An increase in sCr by ≥0.3 mg/dl (≥26.5 μmol/l) within 48 h		
An increase in sCr ≥1.5 times baseline, which is known or presumed to have occurred within the prior 7 days		
UO <0.5 mL/kg h for at least 6 h		
Staging of AKI is done according to the following criteria:		
KDIGO stage	**sCr or eGFR increase**	**Urine output decrease**
1	sCr 1.5–1.9 times baseline *or* 0.3 mg/dl (26.5 μmol/L) increase	<0.5 mL/kg h for 6–12 h
2	sCr 2.0–2.9 times baseline	<0.5 mL/kg h for 12 h
3	sCr 3.0 times baseline *or* Increase in sCr to 4.0 mg/dL (353.6 μmol/L) *or* Initiation of RRT *or* In patients <18 years, decrease in eGFR to <35 mL/min per 1.73 m^2	<0.3 mL/kg h for 24 h *or* Anuria for 12 h

See Ref. [9] for the complete version
sCr serum creatinine, *UO* urine output, *RRT* renal replacement therapy, and *eGFR* estimated glomerular filtration rate. KDIGO guideline is reported in abbreviated form

2.2.3 The KDIGO Defines AKI Using Similar Azotemia and Oliguria Criteria and Includes a GFR Criterion for Patients Younger than 18 Years of Age

In 2003, the Kidney Disease: Improving Global Outcomes (KDIGO) was formed with the aim of implementing clinical practice guidelines for patients with kidney disease. In March 2012, KDIGO published its far-ranging guidelines for the evaluation and management of AKI (Table 2.4) [9].

2.2.4 The US National Kidney Foundation and Others Weigh in on These Three Definitions

A study group of the US National Kidney Foundation, called the NKF-KDOQI (National Kidney Foundation—Kidney Disease Quality Outcome Initiative), reported mixed sentiments about the KDIGO guidelines [12]. The initiative was a group of renal specialists who generally applauded the melding of ADQI, AKIN and KDIGO AKI definitions but was less enthusiastic about the recommendations for AKI management proposed in the KDIGO guidelines. The KDOQI's concern was that many of the management recommendations, though sensible or at least plausible as first-approaches, were unsubstantiated by well-powered controlled clinical studies [12]. Likewise, the Canadian Society of Nephrology (CSN) [13] and the European Renal Best Practices (ERBP) society [14] were hesitant to embrace the KDIGO guideline. By way of the struggle to define and clarify the definition of AKI, and to take the first steps to make the treatment of AKI more evidence-based, much information about the incidence and progression of AKI has been brought to light, even in the absence of any radically new science.

2.2.5 Summary of the Definitions of AKI

The importance of recounting these steps in the evolving definition of AKI is twofold: first, comparing research papers about AKI requires some understanding of the differences between the RIFLE, AKIN, and KDIGO definitions, since they vary in their respective criteria of azotemia, oliguria, estimated glomerular filtration rate (eGFR), and time intervals over which AKI must occur. Secondly, they have different names for each stage of severity. There is yet no consensus on which definition is predominant. The RIFLE acronym [8] is popular in the literature and in medical records, but the KDIGO definition [9, 12] implies future screening and initial management recommendations and is likewise popular. Any of these classifications can be utilized to stratify AKI severity and are used to report incidence and outcome. So far, no one has yet identified a better serum marker than creatinine or better functional criteria than oliguria and GFR to characterize AKI. All three are used one way or another in these three workgroup definitions, for classifying AKI. They are likely all robust and close enough to be reliably used presently.

2.3 The Incidence of AKI

Table 2.5 provides a summary of some relevant publications addressing the incidence of AKI among postoperative and medical inpatients. Various risk factors associated with AKI are also briefly summarized.

Table 2.5 Some studies describing the incidence and risk factors associated with acute kidney injury (AKI)

Study	Type of analysis	*N*	How AKI is defined in the study	Variables associated with AKI	Clinical setting	Main findings
Walsh et al. (2013) [15]	Retrospective	33,330	↑sCr per AKIN definition within 7 days	↓MAP (>55 mmHg)	*Noncardiac surgery* adults	7.4 % pts. developed AKI
Lehman et al. (2010) [18]	Retrospective multivariate logistical regression	16,728	↑sCr per AKIN definition within 48 h	↓MAP (≤80 mmHg) AKI risk related to lowest MAP and duration of ↓BP	*ICU adults*	AKI ↑ for any MAP ≤80 mmHg OR 1.03 (3 %) per each mmHg <80 AKI incidence 50 % for MAP ≤50 mmHg AKI ↑ for each additional hour MAP was decreased below: 70 mmHg (2 %) 60 mmHg (5 %) 50 mmHg (22 %)
Weingarten et al. (2012) [14]	Retrospective case control	9171	↑sCr per AKIN definition within 72 h	↑BMI general anesthesia ↑N of antihypertensive medications CVD PVD DM Transfusion Preoperative anemia	*Major adult orthopedic surgery* Unilateral knee, hip, or shoulder replacement Bilateral knee replacement	AKI developed in 1.82 % Of those with AKI 12.0 % had sCr elevation at 3 months

Kheterpal et al. (2007) [16]	Prospective observational	15,102	CrCl ≤50 mL/min (C&G) within 7 days	Age >59 years ↑BMI, ESLD High-risk surgery PVD COPD	*Noncardiac, general surgery, adult*	0.8 % pts. developed AKI 0.1 % required RRT
Abhela et al. (2009) [17]	Retrospective cohort study; simple binary logistic regression	1166	↑sCr per AKIN definition within 48 h	ASA status RCRI score high-risk surgery ischemic cardiac disease CHF	*ICU adult patients*	7.5 % met AKI criteria
Tujjar et al. (2015) [19]	Retrospective	199	Oliguria within 24 h ↑sCr per AKIN definition within 48 h	Age CKD Higher epinephrine dose In-hospital cardiac arrest hypotension Low admission CrCl High cumulative fluid balance	*Resuscitated cardiac arrest pts., adult*	43 % of pts. developed AKI Pts. with AKI had higher mortality AKI did not predict 3-month neurologic outcome
Harris et al. (2015) [22]	Retrospective	136	RIFLE criteria	Diabetes ↑APACHE III score sepsis	*High-risk adult vascular surgery pts.*, both operative and non-operative management	48 % of pts. developed AKI Pts. with AKI had ↑ short- and long-term mortality and hospital length of stay

(continued)

Table 2.5 (continued)

Study	Type of analysis	*N*	How AKI is defined in the study	Variables associated with AKI	Clinical setting	Main findings
Uchino et al. (2005) [20]	Prospective observational	29,269	ARF defined as oliguria of ≤200 mL in 12 h or BUN ≥84 mg/dL	Causes (%): Sepsis 47.5 Surgery 34.3 CHF 26.9 ↓Vol 25.6 Drug 19.0 Hepatorenal 5.7 Obstructive 2.6 Other 12.2[a]	Pts. admitted to ICUs in multiple countries for *multiple reasons*	5.7 % of pts. developed AKI and 4.3 % needed RRT
Venot et al. (2015) [55]	Case-control	10,911 (3728 sepsis; 510 septic shock)	KDIGO category	55.9 % of septic pts. *without* DM got AKI 72.5 % of septic pts. *with* DM got AKI	*ICU sepsis pts. with or without DM*	Septic pts. *without* DM: 13.8 % had RRT Septic pts. *with* DM: 20.6 % had RRT

AKIN Acute Kidney Injury Network, *Pts.* patients, *OR* odds ratio, *BP* blood pressure, *ARF* acute renal failure, *CKD* chronic kidney disease, *MAP* mean arterial pressure (mmHg), *C&G* Cockcroft and Gault equation for estimating creatinine clearance (CrCl) from serum creatinine (sCr), *BMI* body mass index, *CVD* cerebrovascular disease, *PVD* peripheral vascular disease, *DM* diabetes mellitus, *ESLD* end-stage liver disease, *ASA* American Society of Anesthesiology, *CHF* congestive heart failure/cardiogenic shock, ↓*Vol* intravascular hypovolemia, *BUN* blood urea nitrogen, *RCRI* Revised Cardiac Risk Index

[a]Percentages add to ≥100 % because more than one etiology of AKI might have been listed in Uchino et al. [20]

It is clear from these studies that elective adult patients undergoing planned, especially noncardiac procedures have a lower incidence of AKI as compared to more severely ill categories of patients [14–22]. For example, AKI has been reported to occur in 0.8 % of patients undergoing low-risk surgeries [16], in 1.82 % of patients undergoing orthopedic procedures (shoulder, hip, and knee) [14], and in 7.4 % of patients undergoing any noncardiac intervention [15], while the incidence of AKI is much higher in patients undergoing high-risk (7.5 %) [17] or urgent/emergent surgical procedures (hazard ratio for AKI 1.9 [20]) [15, 16, 18], in ischemic and congestive heart failure patients (hazard ratio for AKI 2.0 [17]), in survivors after cardiac arrest (43 %) [19], in patients admitted to ICU for sepsis (10–20 %) [20, 21], and in both elective or emergent high-risk vascular surgery patients (48 %) [22]. *The greatest risk of AKI is borne by those with preexisting CKD* which is tenfold over the risk of patients who do not have a diagnosis of CKD [23].

2.4 Improving the Diagnosis of AKI: From Creatinine Clearance to the New Biomarkers

Practical assessment of day-to-day kidney function in patients is done implicitly, with simple measurement of UO and sCr, comparing it with a baseline (premorbid) value. According to many authors, however, the benchmark or "gold standard" for measuring renal function is the GFR [24], defined as the amount of blood filtrate per minute emerging from the glomeruli into the proximal tubule lumen, for both kidneys. The practicality of obtaining GFR remains controversial, yet some authors have addressed the complex issue of using serum creatinine as a proxy for actual GFR measurements [25]. Endre et al. [25] noted that the two measurements are not the same, of course, and argued that AKI definitions might do well to avoid GFR criteria. However, they suggested that the estimation of GFR with shorter collection times (e.g., 2–4 h) might indeed be practical and make actual GFR, in association with biomarkers of renal injury, sensitive and feasible on a daily basis. Discussion here will merely address that acceptance of spot sCr and the use of eGFR equations like Cockroft-Gault and MDRD are the nearly universally accepted means of estimating GFR.

Normal GFR, in the absence of CKD, is defined as greater than or equal to 90 mL/min 1.73 m^2 of body surface area (BSA). If CKD has been diagnosed, a patient with a GFR ≥90 mL/min 1.73 m^2 would be said to have KDIGO CKD stage G1. A GFR between 60 and 89 mL/min 1.73 m^2 is said to be mildly decreased (KDIGO stage G2 CKD). Note that this pertains to CKD, not AKI.

2.4.1 The Most Promising Novel Biomarkers of AKI: uAlb/uCr, CysC, NGAL, IL-18, and KIM-1

Though well accepted as a noninvasive marker of GFR, sCr has limitations. It is known to vary with muscle mass, age, gender, liver function, and nonrenal gastrointestinal elimination [26]. Its measurement may be also confounded by exogenous creatinine ingestion. Most importantly, it is well known that sCr is a late indicator of kidney injury [27–29] and that also the reduction in sCr lags as an indicator of improvement in renal function [30]. Moreover, hemodilution may cause a reduction in sCr indicating falsely an improvement in renal function. Finally, its production is decreased in sepsis, unfortunately, just when its use as a marker of AKI makes it a focus of clinical attention [31].

As the need arises to identify AKI earlier and more sensitively than serum creatinine, other biomarkers have been proposed [32]. Table 2.6 shows some features of recently studied biomarkers, including the overall quality of the indicator (i.e., its sensitivity and specificity) as quantitated by its receiver-operator characteristic (ROC) area under the curve (AUC) [33–35]. An AUC value which approaches 1.0 indicates high sensitivity and specificity.

Five of these new biomarkers are among the most promising and will be discussed briefly: urine albumin/creatinine ratio (uAlb/uCr), cystatin-C (CysC), neutrophil gelatinase-associated lipocalin (NGAL), interleukin-18 (IL-18), and kidney injury molecule-1 (KIM-1) [36].

Some authors have merely reexamined the sensitivity and specificity of urine albumin in conjunction with urine creatinine in an attempt to increase the sensitivity and specificity of the two markers, already available in most routine clinical lab panels. Tziakas et al. [29] found the ratio of urinary albumin to creatinine (*uAlb/uCr*) to have a significant predictive value for AKI with an AUC of 0.725, superior to some more modern biomarkers under investigation. Others reported the use of albumin-creatinine ratio as a biomarker of increased risk for cardiovascular morbidity and mortality and all-cause mortality [37].

CysC is a post-gamma-globulin protein first described in 1984 [38]. It belongs to a large class of cysteine proteinase inhibitors. These inhibitors are found in all tissues and bodily fluids, and the enzymes which they inhibit are normally stored in lysozymes produced primarily by nucleated cells throughout the body. It is a small (13 kDa), nonglycosylated, basic protein consisting of 120-amino acid residues [39].

Recent evidence suggests that CysC may be as useful as creatinine or, more so, as a marker for glomerular filtration and AKI. For purposes of assessing renal function, CysC is useful due to its low molecular weight, electrostatic (charge) characteristics, and physical stability: all of these make it easily filtered by the glomerulus. Moreover, its serum concentration is independent of gender, age, or muscle mass, all confounding factors when using creatinine to assess GFR. CysC or the gene coding for it (*CST3*) has also been studied as a biomarker for coronary artery disease [40], congestive heart failure (CHF) [41], squamous cell carcinoma of the head and neck [39], Alzheimer's disease [42, 43], and age-related macular degeneration [43]. This is relevant because the assay for CysC may become more widely used and less expensive and possibly included in clinical laboratory panels in the future.

NGAL, also known as human neutrophil lipocalin (HNL), lipocalin 2, siderocalin, or 24p3, is a small, 25 kDa monomer peptide or a 45 kDa dimer peptide [37]. It is linked covalently with gelatinase (matrix metalloproteinase 9, MMP-9). Its

Table 2.6 Some recent investigations describing novel diagnostic biomarkers of AKI

Study	Type of analysis	Novel biomarker investigated	*N*	Comparison indicator(s)	Setting	AUC (ROC)	Main findings
Tziakis et al. (2015) [29]	Prospective	uNGAL, IL-18, uCysC, pCysC	805	uACR, spot	AKI developing in STEMI and NSTEMI patients	uACR, 0.725	uACR threshold of ≥66.7 μg/mg most accurate, more so than uNGAL or u, pCysC
Hoek et al. (2003) [73]	Prospective cross-sectional analysis	CysC	123	GFR: [^{125}I] iothalamate clearance vs. estimated CysC clearance vs. CrCl (C&G)	Outpatients of a nephrology clinic	CysC, 0.931 C&G, 0.938 Cl, 0.848; both CysC/C&G better than Cl ($p=0.006$) comparison of CysC/C&G, $p=0.815$	Bland-Altman analysis[a] shows that this formula is superior to any other measure in the study[b]: GFR = −4.32 + (80.35/CysC)
Kym et al. (2015) [74]	Prospective cohort study	CysC	85	BUN, sCr, uCr, CysC, CysC-eGFR, AST, LDH, CPK, lactate, myoglobin	Burn patients admitted to ICU	For AKI: LDH, 0.746 lactate, 0.718 sCr, 0.717 CysC, 0.555 For early AKI: LDH, 0.833 sCr, 0.816 AST, 0.790	CysC not useful in predicting AKI in burn patients. LDH, lactate, sCr good LDH, sCr, AST, and Mb good early

(continued)

Table 2.6 (continued)

Study	Type of analysis	Novel biomarker investigated	*N*	Comparison indicator(s)	Setting	AUC (ROC)	Main findings
Stevens et al. (2008) [27]	GFR-estimating equations developed by least squares linear regression. Variables: CysC, sCr, age, sex, race	CysC	3418	GFR: [^{125}I] iothalamate clearance or [^{51}Cr] EDTA clearance vs. sCr/CysC estimated GFR or both	CKD patients	–	CysC alone provides GFR estimates more accurate than sCr alone and nearly as accurate as sCr, age, sex, and race
Nejat et al. (2010) [75]	Prospective	CysC	444	sCr	Pts. admitted to ICUs (with and without preexisting AKI)	sCr, 087 CysC, 0.78 ($p<0.0001$)	In pts. without AKI on ICU admission, the on-entry analyte concentrations were predictive of RRT need (AUC 0.84 for CysC and 0.77 for sCr)
Cruz et al. (2010) [76]	Prospective observational	pNGAL	301	↑sCr (≥50 %) ↓UO (≤0.5 mL/kg h for 6 h)	Adult ICU pts	AKI, 0.78 RRT, 0.82	Correlation of NGAL with AKI severity ($R=0.554$)
Wang et al. (2015) [77]	Prospective cohort study	NGAL	123	NGAL percentile correlation with mortality and MODS	ICU patients with sepsis or septic shock	NGAL predicts mortality (AUC 0.6385)	Mortality 32 % in 12 months
Zhou F (2015) [78]	Meta-analysis	NGAL	4066 (pooled)	NGAL used to predict cardiac surgery-associated AKI	Cardiac surgery pts.	0.86	uNGAL/pNGAL early predictor of AKI especially in neonates/children

Parikh et al. (2013) [52]	Prospective, multicenter cohort study	KIM-1	1219 adults + 319 children	LFABP, NGAL, and composites of the three biomarkers measured at different times	Patients enrolled after cardiac surgery	Adults: urine KIM-1 (6–12 h), 0.78 Children: urine IL-18 (0–6 h) and urine LFABP (from day 2), 0.78	LFABP much more early predictor (6 h) than KIM-1 (2 days)
Nisula et al. (2015) [59]	Prospective cohort study	IL-18	1439	sCr, NGAL	ICU patients	Highest AUC: 0.586 for AKI, 0.667 for stage 3, 0.655 for RRT, 0.536 for 90-day mortality	IL-18 alone felt to be insufficiently accurate
Liu et al. (2013) [79]	Meta-analysis	IL-18	4512 (pooled)	sCr	ICU, ER, cardiac surgery, after contrast	0.70 (overall) 0.68–0.76 (cardiac surgery) 0.62–0.70 (ICU) 0.75–0.82 (children) 0.62–0.70 (adults)	Better predictor of AKI in children than adults, better in cardiac surgery, overall acceptable

Pts. patients, *STEMI/NSTEMI* ST-elevation/non-ST-elevation myocardial infarction, *Mb* myoglobin, *uACR* urine albumin to creatinine ratio, *uCysC/pCysC* urine/plasma cystatin-C, *GFR* glomerular filtration rate (GFR), *C&G* Cockcroft and Gault equation for estimating creatinine clearance (CrCl) from serum creatinine (sCr), *IL-18* interleukin-18, *KIM-1* kidney injury molecule-1, *LFABP* liver fatty acid binding protein, *pNGAL* plasma neutrophil gelatinase-associated lipocalin, *NAG* N-acetyl-β-D-glucosaminidase, *uNGAL* urinary neutrophil gelatinase-associated lipocalin, *uKIM-1* urinary kidney injury molecule-1, *ICU* intensive care unit, *MODS* multi-organ dysfunction syndrome, *ROC* receiver operating characteristic curve, *AUC* area under the curve

[a]Bland-Altman analysis is a statistical test designed to tell if two clinical measurement methods of a single variable are in agreement throughout the range of measurement. It complements the ROC, which is better at comparing various sets of criteria or combinations of tests used in concert to try to establish a binary (i.e., yes-or-no) disease state [80, 81]

[b]The equation estimates GFR in mL/min, using a value of CysC in mg/dL. The most widely used assay is an immune-nephelometric assay with a range of 0.23–7.25 mg/L (17.2–543.0 nmol/L). See Stevens et al. [27]

function is thought to be as a modulator of early inflammation, where it is thought to inhibit bacterial growth, scavenge iron and induce epithelial growth. Plasma NGAL is freely filtered by the glomerulus and then largely reabsorbed by proximal tubular cells. More importantly though, upon renal tubular injury NGAL reabsorption is decreased and NGAL synthesis in epithelial cells of the loop of Henle and of distal tubule segments is strongly upregulated. This makes it an early, sensitive indicator of kidney injury of many etiologies, including diabetic nephropathy [44], ureteral obstruction, nephrotic syndrome and interstitial nephritis, as shown in a variety of animal models and in human disease [45]. It is possible that NGAL might be developed into an early-responding biomarker. In an interesting head-to-head prospective observational study comparing NGAL, CysC, creatinine, and other markers, Ralib et al. [46] measured levels of all these biomarkers beginning at presentation in the emergency room (ER). The study was performed on a small ($n=77$) cohort of patients admitted to the ER with conditions likely to result in AKI (hypotension, ruptured abdominal aortic aneurysm, etc.) and who were followed at very short intervals: 0, 4, 8, and 16 h and 2, 4, and 7 days in the ICU. Of all the biomarkers, only plasma NGAL diagnosed AKI correctly at all time points, including at presentation, and urinary NGAL was best at predicting the composite outcome of mortality or dialysis. Among the sea of candidate biomarkers NGAL merits following as other investigators study it.

IL-18 is a 24 kDa, nonglycosylated polypeptide member of the IL-1β interleukin superfamily of inflammatory cytokines [47]. Its precursor is produced in mononuclear cells in the blood and processed by caspase and then IL-18 is secreted outside the cell to assist in innate and acquired immune responses. This is done by inducing IFN-γ production from T lymphocytes and macrophages and by enhancing cytotoxicity of natural killer [42]. IL-18 is also produced in most endothelial cells of the gastrointestinal tract and kidney (tubular epithelial cells, mesangial cells, and podocytes) [48], thus its potential value as a marker of AKI.

KIM-1 is a larger molecule, a 104 kDa type I transmembrane glycoprotein that contains both an immunoglobulin-like domain and a mucin domain in its extracellular portion [49, 50]. It is expressed at baseline in low levels in healthy proximal tubule cells in the kidney. It is thought to promote apoptotic clearance after ischemia and reperfusion injury of the kidney [49]. Indeed, after kidney ischemia or toxicity, KIM-1 is highly upregulated and released into the extracellular space and urine [49–51], where it is a putative marker of kidney injury.

All these biomarkers have acceptable but not outstanding sensitivities and specificities (AUC values) when used alone (see Table 2.6). An early trend in the literature is of combining two or more biomarkers to increase the composite AUC and thus the overall diagnostic strength of the test [52]. Indeed, a 2014 review of 32 different urine biomarkers, used to predict the progression of acute kidney injury following cardiac surgery, showed that the most sensitive and specific (thus greatest AUC) biomarker was the combination of IL-18 and KIM-1. They had an AUC of 0.93 in predicting an AKIN 3 (RIFLE “F”) stage or death [32].

Which of these new biomarkers will enter into common use (in addition to sCr, which is already widely accepted and embedded in several versions of eGFR equations and should be probably preserved as the standard)? The answer will be determined by the following factors: (1) the biomarker must be excellent in terms of sensitivity and specificity (as measured by AUC) alone or in combination with other biomarkers; (2) it must be fast, leading, not lagging, as a marker (of both onset and recovery of AKI); (3) it must be inexpensive with regard to time, convenience of sampling, labor, ingredients, and assay complexity; (4) it must be accepted by the medical community, the workgroups, and the payers; in other words it must be an acknowledged improvement over the eGFR status quo using sCr; and (5) it must be suitable to health institutions by appearing in an eGFR equation like MDRD; therefore, (6) according to the National Institute of Health (NIH) [53] any candidate biomarker value must be inserted into a so-called IDMS-traceable eGFR equation. An isotope dilution mass spectrometry (IDMS)-traceable equation is an eGFR equation (e.g., MDRD) that is "traceable to" or calibrated by IDMS, an extremely precise means of quantitating GFR. In other words, any eGFR equation must essentially be grounded in creatinine assays that are super-accurate, by way of IDMS calibration.

A detailed discussion of this issue is beyond the scope of this chapter but it is treated exhaustively by Myers et al. [54].

2.5 Outcome Following AKI

As mentioned, a number of published studies (summarized in Table 2.5) addressed the incidence of AKI in various clinical settings, e.g., total joint arthroplasty in elective patients [14], ICU patients [20], cardiology patients monitored for hypotension in the ICU [16], patients with intraoperative hypotension [15], noncardiac general surgery patients with preexisting normal kidney function [18], patients with sepsis or diabetes or both [20, 55, 56], patients resuscitated from cardiac arrest [19], high-risk vascular surgery patients [22], etc. Several authors were able to incorporate long-term outcomes (primarily mortality) in their surveys of AKI patients. Table 2.7 summarizes some of the more widely known studies in which outcome following AKI was examined.

Overall, patients experiencing AKI after surgery have significant increases in mortality. In a very large study including 65,043 patients undergoing major noncardiac surgery, an eightfold increase in 30-day mortality was reported in those who developed postoperative AKI [16]. AKI markedly increases mortality also in ICU patients. Several studies show a clear correlation between the degree of AKI (according to the AKIN and RIFLE criteria) and mortality [57, 58]. In a large retrospective study of 22,303 patients from 22 ICUs, Osterman et al. [57] found a mortality of 10.7 % in patients without AKI, of 20.1 % (odds ratio [OR] 2.59) in those with AKIN stage 1 (RIFLE "R") AKI, of 25.9 % (OR 3.24) in those with stage 2 ("I") AKI, and of 49.6 % (OR 9.38) in those with stage 3 ("F") AKI.

However, an independent association of the various stages of AKI with ICU mortality is harder to demonstrate. In the study by Osterman et al. [57], only AKI stage 3 was independently associated with increased ICU mortality. Stage 2 AKI

Table 2.7 Some recent investigations reporting AKI outcomes

Study	Type of analysis	AKI criteria	N	Comparison indicators	Setting	Important findings
Ricci et al. | (2008) [58]	Meta-analysis	RIFLE	71,000 (pooled)	AKI vs. non-AKI: ICU, hospital, 28-, 30-, 60-, and 90-days mortality	Mostly ICU pts	Pooled OR for death compared to non-AKI: "Risk" 2.40 "Injury" 4.14 "Failure" 6.37
Hildebrand et al. (2015) [82]	Retrospective	AKI needing RRT	188	RRT vs. no RRT need	Parturients cared over a 15-year period	RRT incidence 1/10,000 Among those needing RRT: 4.3 % died 3.9 % on RRT 4 months later
Uchino et al. (2005) [20]	Prospective observational	↑sCr per AKIN definition within 48 h	29,269	AKI vs. non-AKI:	ICU pts.	Pts. who developed AKI had higher SAPS II and APACHE II scores and higher ICU, hospital, and 6-months mortality AKI was an independent risk factor for hospital mortality (OR 3.12, 95 % CI 1.41–6.93, $P=0.005$)
Rimes-Stigare et al. (2015) [83]	Prospective observational	RRT or ↑sCr (×1.5) or sCr ≥4.0 mg/dL (354 μmol/L)	97,782 (5273 with AKI)	Patients who had AKI were more likely to die (MRR 2.87)	ICU pts.	20 % of AKI pts. were dead within 4 days AKI survivors had a 7-fold ↑risk of developing CKD and a 22-fold ↑ risk of ESRD compared with non-AKI pts

Osterman et al. (2008) [57]	Retrospective	↑sCr per RIFLE criteria or need for RRT	22,303 (7898 with AKI)	AKI vs. non-AKI	ICU patients without preexisting CKD	ICU mortality (OR) 10.7 % without AKI (1.0) 20.1 % "risk" (2.59) 25.9 % "injury" (3.24) 49.6 % "failure" (9.38) Only AKI-"failure" was independently associated with ICU mortality AKI-"injury" not associated with mortality AKI-"risk" associated with a reduced risk of mortality (see text)
Nisula et al. (2013) [84]	Prospective multicenter study	KDIGO criteria	1568 (635 with AKI)	Follow-up at 6 months of AKI pts. admitted to ICU vs. ICU pts. without AKI	ICU pts.	35.3 % of pts. with AKI as compared to 16.5 % of pts. without AKI were died within six months AKI patients had lower quality-of-life indices six months later

Pts. patients *ICU* intensive care unit, *OR* odds ratio ,*CI* confidence interval, *AKI* acute kidney injury, *RRT* renal replacement therapy, *MRR* mortality rate ratio, *CKD* chronic kidney disease, *ESRD* end-stage renal disease

was not independently associated with increased ICU mortality. Surprisingly, stage 1 AKI and RRT were independently associated with reduced ICU mortality. The authors acknowledged that because AKIN criteria allowed including all patients on RRT as AKI stage 3, and because some 583 persons began to receive RRT before their AKI had actually progressed to AKI stage 3, the picture may be confused.

The 6-month outcomes of surviving AKI patients in a large Finnish study using the KDIGO AKI definition have been recently reported [59]. Among 933 patients studied, 224 patients (35.3 %) with AKI died within 6 months, as compared with 154 (16.5 %) patients without AKI. Surviving AKI patients had lower quantitative quality-of-life indices 6 months later, as opposed to those who did not have AKI. Surprisingly though, their self-reported assessments of well-being were equivalent to survivors without AKI.

2.6 Summary and Discussion

The reexamination of AKI from a standpoint of its definition, classification, and diagnosis began around 2000 when the first definitions of AKI were propounded.

Paired with improvements in the definition of AKI was the problem of how to diagnose it. The traditional, "gold standard" methods (clearances of various inert compounds such as phenol red and inulin) had long ago evolved to more practical spot assays of serum creatinine and albumin. The problems with creatinine are, however, that it is a late (24–48 h), indirect indicator of kidney injury [27, 28], and that its production times are impaired in sepsis (a high-risk condition for the kidney) [60] and they also decrease in cachexia or extremes of age.

From this conundrum came a new starting point. Better understanding of AKI has led to discrimination between the various mechanisms of kidney injury. Apart from preexisting CKD [2, 23], sepsis is the most powerful risk factor in developing AKI [20, 56, 61, 62]. As a rule, AKI will develop predictably in about 19 % of patients with "moderate" sepsis (fever or hypothermia with infection, tachycardia, tachypnea, and leukocytosis), 23 % of patients with severe sepsis (the above plus lactatemia, oliguria, or mental status changes), and 51 % of patients with septic shock (all the above plus systolic blood pressure less than 90 mmHg after fluid resuscitation) when blood cultures are positive [56, 62, 63]. Better knowledge about this type of kidney injury may lead to better diagnosis of at-risk patients and more rapid therapy of sepsis. Likewise better biomarker-led diagnosis of septic AKI might result in intervention hours or days before azotemia or oliguria develop. Novel biomarkers, such as IL-18, are differentially sensitive to AKI caused by different mechanisms. IL-18 is thought to increase in early (3 h) sepsis-induced AKI as opposed to a slower rise in AKI from ischemia in hypotensive states [61, 64, 65]. Indeed, it is thought that the pathophysiological mechanisms for AKI from sepsis or non-septic etiologies (e.g., ischemia) are completely different [61]. With research targeted at the most harmful intermediaries in the septic process, therapeutic or preventative drugs or biologics may be found to protect the kidney in systemic inflammatory response syndrome (SIRS) and sepsis.

Other approaches might prevent or mitigate AKI in patients at risk for renal ischemia. As shown in the papers by Lehman et al. [18], Osterman et al. [57], and Raimundo et al. [66], huge databases of ICU time-series blood pressure readings and other clinical data have been mined to show the most sensitive criterion for adequate perfusion of the kidney in ICU and surgical patients. The time-honored 90 mmHg systolic threshold may soon, in routine clinical practice, be replaced by the more sensitive and specific 55 mmHg mean pressure as the commonly taught threshold for immediate intervention with vasopressor medication or fluids. Other hemodynamic and respiratory factors appear to contribute to the risk of AKI with unclear mechanisms: obesity, hyperuricemia, low indexed systemic oxygen delivery, hyperlactatemia, elevated central venous pressure, and the use of mechanical ventilation have been shown to be important but ill-defined factors [57, 66].

The ischemia-reperfusion paradigm so widely invoked in studies of stroke and myocardial infarction may likewise provide a framework for studying AKI from causes other than sepsis. However, it is generally felt that AKI from sepsis (but also, e.g., after cardiopulmonary bypass) is via other, largely inflammatory pathways. Accordingly, the mere restoration or improvement of renal perfusion will be insufficient to reverse kidney damage [67]. Other authors, using a combinatorial systems biology and proteomic approach, have identified the glutaminergic signaling pathway, induced by overactivation of *N*-methyl-D-aspartate receptors, as perhaps the inciting factor in AKI [68].

Lastly, bioinformatics approaches enable wide surveys of thousands of genes [69, 70] that are activated or repressed in AKI, as well as epigenetic changes that occur with AKI [71]. New candidate gene products and pathways discovered from this research will, it is hoped, open avenues to explore and to better prevent and mitigate AKI in the future.

References

1. Chawla LS, Amdur RL, Shaw AD et al (2014) The association between AKI and long-term renal and cardiovascular outcomes in United States veterans. Clin J Am Soc Nephrol 9:448–456
2. Go AS, Chertow GM, Fan D et al (2004) Chronic kidney disease and the risks of death, cardiovascular events, and hospitalization. N Eng J Med 351:1296–1305
3. Lafrance JP, Miller DR (2010) Acute kidney injury associates with increased long-term mortality. J Am Soc Nephrol 21:345–352
4. James MT, Ghali WA, Knudtson ML et al (2011) Associations between acute kidney injury and cardiovascular and renal outcomes after coronary angiography. Circulation 123:409–416
5. Tsagalis G, Akrivos T, Alevizaki M et al (2009) Renal dysfunction in acute stroke: an independent predictor of long-term all combined vascular events and overall mortality. Nephrol Dial Transplant 24:194–200
6. Farley SJ (2007) Acute kidney injury/acute renal failure: standardizing nomenclature, definitions and staging. Nat Clin Pract Nephrol 3:405

7. Niessenson AR (1998) Acute renal failure: definition and pathogenesis. Kidney Int Suppl 66:S7–S10
8. Bellomo R, Ronco C, Kellum JA et al (2004) Acute renal failure—definition, outcome measures, animal models, fluid therapy and information technology needs: the Second International Consensus Conference of the Acute Dialysis Quality Initiative (ADQI) Group. Crit Care 8:R204–R212
9. Kidney Disease: Improving Global Outcomes (KDIGO) Acute Kidney Injury Work Group (2012) KDIGO clinical practice guideline for acute kidney injury. Kidney Int Suppl 2:1–138
10. Ronco C, Kellum JA, Mehta R (2001) Acute dialysis quality initiative (ADQI). Nephrol Dial Transplant 16(8):1555–1558
11. Molitoris BA, Levin A, Warnock DG et al (2007) Improving outcomes of acute kidney injury: report of an initiative. Nat Clin Pract Nephrol 3:439–442
12. Palevsky PM, Liu KD, Brophy PD et al (2013) KDOQI US commentary on the 2012 KDIGO clinical practice guideline for acute kidney injury. Am J Kidney Dis 6:649–672
13. Fliser D, Laville M, Covic A et al (2012) A European Renal Best Practice (ERBP) position statement on the Kidney Disease Improving Global Outcomes (KDIGO) clinical practice guidelines on acute kidney injury: part 1: definitions, conservative management and contrast induced nephropathy. Nephrol Dial Transplant 27:4263–4272
14. Weingarten TN, Gurrieri C, Jarett PD et al (2012) Acute kidney injury following total joint arthroplasty: retrospective analysis. Can J Anaesth 59(12):1111–1118
15. Walsh M, Devereaux PJ, Garg AX et al (2013) Relationship between intraoperative mean arterial pressure and clinical outcomes after noncardiac surgery. Anesthesiology 119:1–9
16. Kheterpal S, Tremper KK, Englesbe MJ et al (2007) Predictors of postoperative acute renal failure after noncardiac surgery in patients with previously normal renal function. Anesthesiology 107:892–902
17. Abhela FJ, Botelho M, Fernandes V et al (2009) Determinants of postoperative acute kidney injury. Crit Care 13:R79
18. Lehman LW, Saeed M, Moody G, Mark R (2010) Hypotension as a risk factor for acute kidney injury in ICU patients. Comput Cardiol 37:1095–1098
19. Tujjar O, Mineo G, Dell'Anna A et al (2015) Acute kidney injury after cardiac arrest. Crit Care 19:169
20. Uchino S, Kellum JA, Bellomo R et al (2005) Acute renal failure in critically ill patients: a multinational, multicenter study. JAMA 294:813–818
21. Honore PM, Jacobs R, Hendrickx I et al (2015) Prevention and treatment of sepsis-induced acute kidney injury: an update. Ann Intensive Care 5:51
22. Harris DG, Koo G, McCrone MP et al (2015) Acute kidney injury in critically ill vascular surgery patients is common and associated with increased mortality. Front Surg 2:8
23. Chawla LS, Eggers PW, Star RA et al (2014) Acute kidney injury and chronic kidney disease as interconnected syndromes. N Eng J Med 371:58–66
24. Kidney Disease: Improving Global Outcomes (KDIGO) CKD Workgroup (2013) KDIGO 2012 clinical practice guideline for the evaluation and management of chronic kidney disease. Kidney Int Suppl 3:1–150
25. Endre ZH, Pickering JW, Walker RJ (2001) Clearance and beyond: the complementary roles of GFR measurement and injury biomarkers in acute kidney injury (AKI). Am J Physiol Renal Physiol 301:F697–F707
26. Shemesh O, Golbetz H, Kriss JP et al (1985) Limitations of creatinine as a filtration marker in glomerulopathic patients. Kidney Int 28:830–838
27. Stevens LA, Coresh J, Schmid CH et al (2008) Estimating GFR using serum cystatin C alone and in combination with serum creatinine: a pooled analysis of 3418 individuals with CKD. Am J Kidney Dis 51:395–406
28. Dai X, Zeng Z, Fu C et al (2015) Diagnostic value of neutrophil gelatinase-associated lipocalin, cystatin C, and soluble triggering receptor expressed on myeloid cells-1 in critically ill patients with sepsis-associated acute kidney injury. Crit Care 19:223

29. Tziakas D, Chalikias G, Kareli D et al (2015) Spot urine albumin to creatinine ratio outperforms novel acute kidney injury biomarkers in patients with acute myocardial infarction. Int J Cardiol 197:48–55
30. Vaidya VS, Ramirez V, Ichimura T et al (2006) Urinary kidney injury molecule-1: a sensitive quantitative biomarker for early detection of kidney tubular injury. Am J Physiol Renal Physiol 290:F517–F529
31. Doi K, Yuen PS, Eisner C et al (2009) Reduced production of creatinine limits its use as a marker of kidney injury in sepsis. J Am Soc Nephrol 20:1217–1221
32. Arthur JM, Hill EG, Alge JL et al (2014) Evaluation of 32 urine biomarkers to predict the progression of acute kidney injury after cardiac surgery. Kidney Int 85:431–438
33. Bamber D (1975) The area above the ordinal dominance graph and the area below the receiver operating characteristic curve. J Math Psychol 12:387–415
34. Hanley JA, McNeil BJ (1982) The meaning and use of the area under a receiver operating characteristic (ROC) curve. Radiology 143:29–36
35. Zweig MH, Campbell G (1993) Receiver-operating characteristic (ROC) plots: a fundamental evaluation tool in clinical medicine. Clin Chem 39:561–577
36. Ferguson MA, Vaidya V, Bonventre JV (2008) Biomarkers of nephrotoxic acute kidney injury. Toxicology 245:182–193
37. Vart P, Scheven L, Lambers Heerspink HJ et al (2016) Urine albumin-creatinine ratio versus albumin excretion for albuminuria staging: a prospective longitudinal cohort study. Am J Kidney Dis 67(1):70–78
38. Brzin J, Popovic T, Turk V et al (1984) Human cystatin, a new protein inhibitor of cysteine proteinases. Biochem Biophys Res Commun 118:103–109
39. Strojan P, Oblak I, Svetic B et al (2004) Cysteine proteinase inhibitor cystatin C in squamous cell carcinoma of the head and neck: relation to prognosis. Br J Cancer 90:1961–1968
40. Kiyosue A, Hirata Y, Ando J et al (2010) Plasma cystatin C concentration reflects the severity of coronary artery disease in patients without chronic kidney disease. Circ J 74:2441–2447
41. Ruan ZB, Zhu L, Yin YG et al (2014) Cystatin C, N-terminal probrain natriuretic peptides and outcomes in acute heart failure with acute kidney injury in a 12-month follow-up: insights into the cardiorenal syndrome. J Res Med Sci 19:404–409
42. Kaur G, Levy E (2012) Cystatin C in Alzheimer's disease. Front Mol Neurosci 5:79
43. Butler JM, Umar Sharif U, Ali M et al (2015) A missense variant in CST3 exerts a recessive effect on susceptibility to age-related macular degeneration resembling its association with Alzheimer's disease. Hum Genet 2015 134(7):705–715
44. Liu F, Yang H, Chen H et al (2015) High expression of neutrophil gelatinase-associated lipocalin (NGAL) in the kidney proximal tubules of diabetic rats. Adv Med Sci 60:133–138
45. Kuwabara T, Mori K, Mukoyama M et al (2009) Urinary neutrophil gelatinase-associated lipocalin levels reflect damage to glomeruli, proximal tubules, and distal nephrons. Kidney Int 75:285–294
46. Ralib A, Pickering JW, Shaw GM et al (2014) The clinical utility window for acute kidney injury biomarkers in the critically ill. Crit Care 18:601
47. Okamura H, Tsutsui H, Toshinori K et al (1995) Cloning of a new cytokine that induces IFN-γ production by T cells. Nature 378:88–91
48. Yano T, Nozaki Y, Kinoshita K et al (2015) The pathological role of IL-18Rα in renal ischemia/reperfusion injury. Lab Invest 95:78–91
49. Ichimura T, Bonventre JV, Bailly V et al (1998) Kidney injury molecule-1 (KIM-1), a putative epithelial cell adhesion molecule containing a novel immunoglobulin domain, is up-regulated in renal cells after injury. J Biol Chem 273:4135–4142
50. Bailly V, Zhang Z, Meier W et al (2002) Shedding of kidney injury molecule-1, a putative adhesion protein involved in renal regeneration. J Biol Chem 277:39739–39748
51. Zwiers AJM, de Wildt SN, vanRosmalen J et al (2015) Urinary neutrophil gelatinase-associated lipocalin identifies critically ill young children with acute kidney injury following intensive care admission: a prospective cohort study. Crit Care 19:181

52. Parikh CR, Thiessen-Philbrook H, Garg AX et al (2013) Performance of kidney injury molecule-1 and liver fatty acid-binding protein and combined biomarkers of AKI after cardiac surgery. Clin J Am Soc Nephrol 8:1079–1088
53. http://www.niddk.nih.gov/health-information/health-communication-programs/nkdep/lab-evaluation/gfr/creatinine-standardization/recommendations/Pages/recommendations.aspx. Webpage accessed 22 Jan 2016
54. Myers GL, Miller WG, Coresh J et al (2006) Recommendations for improving serum creatinine measurement: a report from the Laboratory Working Group of the National Kidney Disease Education Program. Clin Chem 52(1):5–18
55. Venot M, Weis L, Clec'h C et al (2015) Acute kidney injury in severe sepsis and septic shock in patients with and without diabetes mellitus: a multicenter study. PLoS One 10(5):e0127411
56. Rangel-Frausto MS, Pittet D, Costigan M et al (1995) The natural history of the systemic inflammatory response syndrome (SIRS): a prospective study. JAMA 273:117–123
57. Osterman M, Chang R, Riyadh ICU Program Users Group (2008) Correlation between the AKI classification and outcome. Crit Care 12:R144
58. Ricci Z, Cruz D, Ronco C (2008) The RIFLE criteria and mortality in acute kidney injury: a systematic review. Kidney Int 73:538–546
59. Nisula S, Yang R, Poukkanen M et al (2015) Predictive value of urine interleukin-18 in the evolution and outcome of acute kidney injury in critically ill adult patients. Br J Anaesth 114:460–468
60. Umbro I, Gentile G, Tinti F et al (2016) Recent advances in pathophysiology and biomarkers of sepsis-induced acute kidney injury. J Infect 72(2):131–142
61. Zarjou A, Agarwal A (2011) Sepsis and acute kidney injury. J Am Soc Nephrol 22:999–1006
62. Schrier RW, Wang W (2004) Acute renal failure and sepsis. N Engl J Med 351:159–169
63. Riedemann NC, Guo RF, Ward PA (2003) The enigma of sepsis. J Clin Invest 112:460–467
64. Bellomo R, Bagshaw S, Langenberg C, Ronco C (2007) Pre-renal azotemia: a flawed paradigm in critically ill septic patients? Contrib Nephrol 156:1–9
65. Bagshaw SM, Langenberg C, Haase M et al (2007) Urinary biomarkers in septic acute kidney injury. Intensive Care Med 33:1285–1296
66. Raimundo M, Crichton S, Syed Y et al (2016) Low systemic oxygen delivery and BP and risk of progression of early AKI. Clin J Am Soc Nephrol 10(8):1340–1349
67. Landoni G, Baiardo Redaelli M, Pisano A (2016) Dopamine derivatives and acute kidney injury: the search for the magic bullet continues … and leads to new (magic?) targets. Nephrol Dial Transplant 31(4):512–514
68. Husi H, Sanchez-Nino MD, Delles C et al (2013) A combinatorial approach of proteomics and system biology in unravelling the mechanisms of acute kidney injury (AKI): involvement of NMDA receptor GRIN1 in murine AKI. BMC Syst Biol 7:110
69. Boyd JH, McConechy M, Walley KR (2014) Acute organ injury is associated with alterations in the cell-free plasma transcriptome. Intensive Care Med Exp 2:7
70. Stafford-Smith M, Li YJ, Mathew JP et al (2015) Genome-wide association study of acute kidney injury after coronary bypass graft surgery identifies susceptibility loci. Kidney Int 88(4):823–832
71. Tang J, Zhuang S (2015) Epigenetics in acute kidney injury. Curr Opin Nephrol Hypertens 24:351–358
72. Mehta RL, Kellum JA, Shah SV et al (2007) Acute Kidney Injury Network: report of an initiative to improve outcomes in acute kidney injury. Crit Care 11(2):R31
73. Hoek FJ, Kemperman AW, Krediet RT (2003) A comparison between cystatin C, plasma creatinine and the Cockcroft and Gault formula for the estimation of glomerular filtration rate. Nephrol Dial Transplant 18:2024–2031
74. Kym D, Cho YS, Yoon J et al (2015) Evaluation of diagnostic biomarkers for acute kidney injury in major burn patients. Ann Surg Treat Res 88:281–288
75. Nejat M, Pickering JW, Walker RJ et al (2010) Rapid detection of acute kidney injury by plasma cystatin C in the intensive care unit. Nephrol Dial Transplant 25:3283–3289

76. Cruz DN, deCal M, Garzotto F et al (2010) Plasma neutrophil gelatinase-associated lipocalin is an early biomarker for acute kidney injury in an adult ICU population. Intensive Care Med 36:444–451
77. Wang B, Chen G, Zhang J et al (2015) Increased neutrophil gelatinase-associated lipocalin is associated with mortality and multiple organ dysfunction syndrome in severe sepsis and septic shock. Shock 44:234–238
78. Zhou F, Luo Q, Wang L, Han L (2016) Diagnostic value of neutrophil gelatinase-associated lipocalin for early diagnosis of cardiac surgery-associated acute kidney injury: a meta-analysis. Eur J Cardiothorac Surg 49(3):746–755
79. Liu Y, Guo W, Zhang J et al (2013) Urinary interleukin 18 for detection of acute kidney injury: a meta-analysis. Am J Kidney Dis 62:1058–1067
80. Bland JM, Altman DG (1986) Statistical methods for assessing agreement between two methods of clinical measurement. Lancet 1(8476):307–310
81. Altman DG, Bland JM (1983) Measurement in medicine: the analysis of method comparison studies. The Statistician 32:307–317
82. Hildebrand AM, Liu K, Shariff SZ et al (2015) Characteristics and outcomes of AKI treated with dialysis during pregnancy and the postpartum period. J Am Soc Nephrol 26(12):3085–3091
83. Rimes-Stigare C, Frumento P, Bottai M et al (2015) Evolution of chronic renal impairment and long-term mortality after de novo acute kidney injury in the critically ill: a Swedish multicentre cohort study. Crit Care 19:221
84. Nisula S, Vaara ST, Kaukonen KM et al (2013) Six-month survival and quality of life of intensive care patients with acute kidney injury. Crit Care 17:R250

3 Reducing Mortality in Acute Kidney Injury: The Democracy-Based Approach to Consensus

Massimiliano Greco, Margherita Pintaudi, and Antonio Pisano

3.1 Introduction

Evidence-based medicine (EBM) is the cornerstone of medical epistemology. This "movement," which was born more than three decades ago, has promoted a critical revision of the clinical and scientific medical knowledge. However, the EBM approach is not free from limitations [1], and this was demonstrated in particular in the field of intensive care medicine [2].

Internal validity and generalizability of randomized clinical trials (RCTs) are limited in the intensive care setting [3, 4] due to the complexity of clinical conditions and therapeutic interventions to be investigated (and accordingly the frequent lack of "conventional" therapies to be used as control), the large amount and wide variability of concomitant treatments, and difficulties in definition of end points (with large use of composite end points) [5]. A "pendulum effect" has been proposed to define the sequence of opposite results in clinical trials [2].

Guidelines and consensus conferences have been introduced as a simple tool to summarize scientific evidences and to ensure optimal care to patients, while helping clinicians to achieve best practice in their daily clinical management. A controversy on a debated topic is normally settled by the opinion of experts in the field. This strategy, however, is not only far from the ideal approach of EBM epistemology but is being increasingly criticized for the risk of introducing expert opinion biases [6].

M. Greco, MD (✉) • M. Pintaudi
Department of Anesthesia and Intensive Care, San Raffaele Scientific Institute, via Olgettina 60, Milan 20132, Italy
e-mail: greco.massimiliano@hsr.it; margherita.pintaudi@gmail.com

A. Pisano
Cardiac Anesthesia and Intensive Care Unit, A.O.R.N. "Dei Colli", Monaldi Hospital, via L. Bianchi, Naples 80131, Italy
e-mail: antoniopisanoMD@libero.it

© Springer International Publishing Switzerland 2016

G. Landoni et al. (eds.), *Reducing Mortality in Acute Kidney Injury*,
DOI 10.1007/978-3-319-33429-5_3

A new method to achieve consensus on medical evidence has been recently developed and already employed in various settings [8, 9] in the attempt to overcome some limits and, possibly, to improve the reliability of "classic" consensus conferences [7]. This approach has the advantage of sharing the best available evidence with a worldwide audience of clinicians, to allow them to discuss on it and propose further evidence, and to reach a final consensus through a democratic process.

This method has been also applied in the recent first international consensus conference conducted to identify the interventions (drugs, techniques, or strategies) with a statistical significant effect on mortality in critically ill patients with, or at risk for, acute kidney injury (AKI) [10]. The process of consensus building is outlined in Fig. 3.1 and is fully described in the following sections.

3.2 The Process of Consensus Building

3.2.1 Systematic Literature Research

A systematic literature research was performed to identify any intervention influencing mortality in critically patients with AKI. PubMed, Embase, BioMed Central,

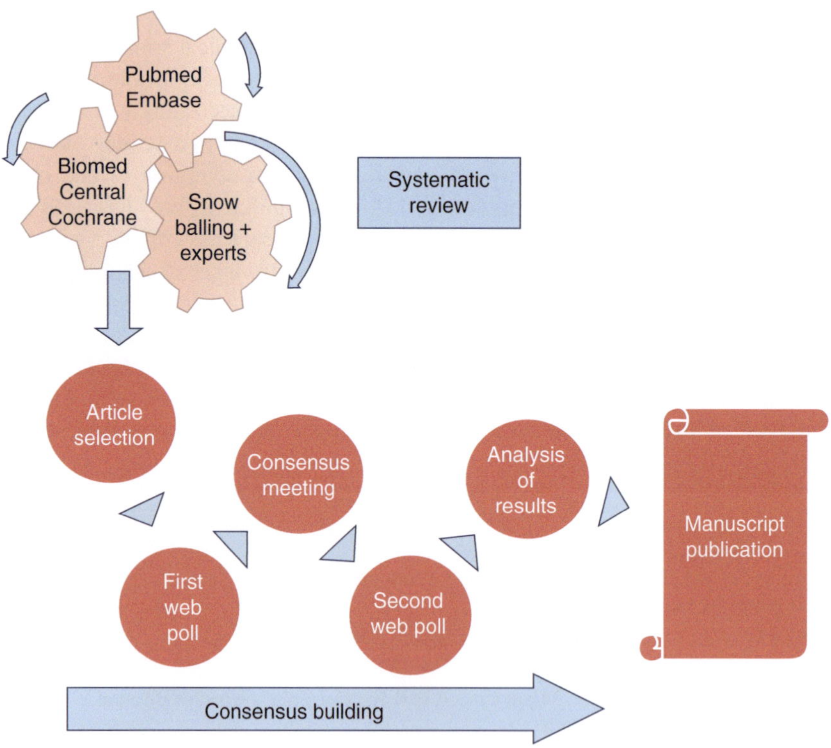

Fig. 3.1 The democracy-based consensus process

and the Cochrane Library were searched without time limits, using the search strategy reported in Box 3.1. Further topics were proposed by a group of experts and by snowballing, i.e., backward cross-checking of article references. Any paper on critically ill patients with or at risk for AKI, published in a peer-reviewed journal, was included if reporting a statistically significant effect on mortality ($p<0.05$) at any end point. A conservative strategy was employed to avoid exclusion of any relevant article in this phase.

Box 3.1. PubMed Search Strategy

((acute AND (renal OR kidney) AND (failure OR injury)) OR (renal AND replacement AND therapy)) AND ((death* OR survival OR mortality)) AND (prevent* OR reducti* OR reduci*) AND (significat* OR significan*) AND (randomized controlled trial[pt] OR controlled clinical trial[pt] OR randomized controlled trials[mh] OR random allocation[mh] OR double-blind method[mh] OR single-blind method[mh] OR clinical trial[pt] OR clinical trials[mh] OR (clinical trial[tw] OR ((singl*[tw] OR doubl*[tw] OR trebl*[tw] OR tripl*[tw]) AND (mask*[tw] OR blind[tw])) OR (latin square[tw]) OR placebos[mh] OR placebo*[tw] OR random*[tw] OR research design[mh:noexp] OR comparative study[tw] OR follow-up studies[mh] OR prospective studies[mh] OR cross-over studies[mh] OR control*[tw] OR prospectiv*[tw] OR volunteer*[tw]) NOT (animal[mh] NOT human[mh]))

A total of 691 papers were analyzed as full text, and 657 were excluded due to the lack of inclusion criteria. Therefore, 34 papers were selected for further inclusion in the consensus process.

3.2.2 Global Voting and International Consensus Meeting

The topics of these 34 studies were subjected to a first worldwide evaluation via web polling. In the period between January 1, 2012, and February 14, 2012, a website allowed to vote in favor or against the selected topics. Moreover, participants were allowed to suggest online other interventions or relevant literature.

On February 14, 2012, a core group of experienced clinicians of various disciplines (including intensivists, anesthesiologists, and nephrologists) met at the Vita-Salute San Raffaele University (Milan, Italy) to discuss the identified papers and topics, as well as the results of the first web voting. Topics were introduced to the meeting audience by a discussant and then evaluated on:

1. The completeness of the literature review, including most recent evidence
2. The type and quality of scientific evidence supporting the influence on mortality (RCTs, meta-analyses, case-matched studies, or other)
3. The study population of included articles, to assess if it was derived entirely or partially from patients with or at risk for AKI

After thorough discussion, a position statement was produced for each topic, summarizing the intervention, the reason for its inclusion, and the challenges in evaluation, if any. Each statement also reported a recommendation, which was rated according to the grade classification on strength and quality of evidence (Table 3.1) [11]. According to the grade classification, the strength of the recommendation is defined by one of two numbers: (1) represents a strong recommendation, while (2) represents a suggestion or weak recommendation. A letter among A, B, and C indicates the quality of evidence for the recommendation, according to the type of studies from which evidence is derived:

- Level A: RCTs without important limitations or overwhelming evidences from observational studies (high-quality evidence)
- Level B: RCTs with important limitations or exceptionally strong evidence from observational studies (moderate-quality evidence)
- Level C: observational studies or case series (low-quality evidence)

Five topics were excluded during the consensus meeting, due to the lack of information or evidence about critically ill patients with or at risk for AKI.

Table 3.1 Grade of recommendation for the 18 identified interventions.

Grade of recommendation	Intervention
1A	None
1B	Albumin in cirrhotic patients
	Hydroxyethyl starch (*avoid*)
1C	Perioperative hemodynamic optimization
	Terlipressin in hepatorenal syndrome type 1
2A	None
2B	Fenoldopam[a]
	Periangiography hemofiltration
2C	Citrate in continuous RRT
	CVVH in severely burned patients
	Continuous RRT
	Early RRT
	Furosemide by continuous infusion
	Human Immunoglobulin
	Increased intensity of RRT
	Loop diuretics (*avoid*)
	N-acetylcysteine
	Plasma exchange in multiple myeloma-associated AKI
	Positive fluid balance (*avoid*)
	Vasopressin in septic shock

RRT renal replacement therapy
[a]Probably no longer to be recommended (see Chap. 13)

Fifteen interventions which were shown to increase survival, and three that might increase mortality, were finally identified during the consensus meeting. These 18 interventions, supported overall by 25 papers [12–36], are reported in Table 3.2.

3.2.3 Global Appraisal of Consensus Statements

Between February 15, 2012 and April 1, 2012, the second web poll was conducted. The consensus website hosted the poll on the topics and the recommendations thereon, which were issued during the Milan consensus meeting. A large cohort of participants, including the first web voters and the participants to the consensus meeting, were invited to vote if they agreed or not with interventions and recommendations. Moreover, voters could express on a Likert scale ("definitely," "probably yes," "don't know," "probably not," "definitely not") if they would follow these recommendations in their clinical practice. Multiple voting was prevented through registration of e-mail address, and all participants were asked to declare any relevant conflict of interest.

3.2.4 Consensus Final Results

A total of 311 participants from 62 different countries took part in the Democratic Consensus Conference. After the final web poll, data were analyzed and results were made available to the authors.

Table 3.2 The 18 interventions affecting mortality identified by the democracy-based consensus process

Increasing survival	Increasing mortality
Perioperative hemodynamic optimization [12]	Positive fluid balance [13, 14]
Albumin in cirrhotic patients [15, 16]	Hydroxyethyl starch [16, 17]
Terlipressin in hepatorenal syndrome type 1 [18]	Loop diuretics [19]
Human immunoglobulin [20]	
Periangiography hemofiltration [21]	
Fenoldopam [22]	
Plasma exchange in multiple myeloma-associated AKI [23]	
Increased intensity of RRT [24–26]	
CVVH in severely burned patients [27]	
Vasopressin in septic shock [28, 29]	
Furosemide by continuous infusion [30]	
Citrate in continuous RRT [31]	
N-acetylcysteine [32, 33]	
Continuous RRT [34]	
Early RRT [35, 36]	

The agreement between global polling and consensus meeting recommendations was high in most topics. However, there were several topics (plasma exchange in multiple myeloma, vasopressin in septic shock, furosemide by continuous infusion, citrate in continuous renal replacement therapy, *N*-acetyl-cysteine, and loop diuretics) for which the agreement was significantly lower among web voters than among consensus meeting participants.

The 18 selected topics with a significant impact on survival in critically ill patients with AKI, the consensus statements, and the results of the web survey were included in a paper recently published as a special article in the *Journal of Cardiothoracic and Vascular Anesthesia* [10].

Conclusion

This was the first International Consensus Conference on mortality reduction in critically ill patients with or at risk for AKI, and it was conducted through the new idea of democracy-based medicine. The are several advantages with this approach: (a) the consensus conference is grounded on a full systematic review of the available literature, conducted ex novo and fully updated; (b) it includes the opinion of experts, but it overcomes the limitations of a "classic" consensus conference conducted by experts only, as it includes a double global voting that allows for a democratic assessment of recommendations; and (c) it allows to highlight the gap between the "theory" from literature evidence and the daily clinical practice reported by respondents.

The democracy-based consensus process identified a total of 18 interventions (drugs/techniques/strategies) with a significant impact on survival in critically ill patients with or at risk for AKI: 15 interventions have been shown to increase survival and 3 might increase mortality. A graded recommendation was provided for all of them.

The following 18 chapters of this book (Chaps. 4, 5, 6, 7, 8, 9, 10, 11, 12, 13, 14, 15, 16, 17, 18, 19, 20, and 21) will unfold the main evidences, general principles, pharmacological/pathophysiological aspects, and therapeutic use of each of the identified interventions, providing the reader with a valuable resource to guide his/her clinical practice and opening the door for future lines of research.

Finally, an updated review of papers dealing with interventions which may significantly affect mortality in AKI patients, identified after the consensus process according to the same search strategy, is reported in Chap. 22.

References

1. Ashcroft RE (2004) Current epistemological problems in evidence based medicine. J Med Ethics 30(2):131–135
2. Vincent J-L (2010) We should abandon randomized controlled trials in the intensive care unit. Crit Care Med 38(10 Suppl):S534–S538
3. Webb SAR (2015) Putting critical care medicine on trial. Crit Care Med 43(8):1767–1768

4. Sevransky JE (2015) Known unknowns. Crit Care Med 43(8):1557–1558
5. Grasselli G, Gattinoni L, Kavanagh B et al (2007) Feasibility, limits and problems of clinical studies in Intensive Care Unit. Minerva Anestesiol 73(11):595–601
6. Baur X, Budnik LT, Ruff K et al (2015) Ethics, morality, and conflicting interests: how questionable professional integrity in some scientists supports global corporate influence in public health. Int J Occup Environ Health 37(1):172–175
7. Greco M, Zangrillo A, Mucchetti M et al (2015) Democracy-based consensus in medicine. J Cardiothorac Vasc Anesth 29(2):506–509
8. Landoni G, Rodseth RN, Santini F et al (2012) Randomized evidence for reduction of perioperative mortality. J Cardiothorac Vasc Anesth 26(5):764–772
9. Landoni G, Comis M, Conte M et al (2015) Mortality in multicenter critical care trials: an analysis of interventions with a significant effect. Crit Care Med 43(8):1559–1568
10. Landoni G, Bove T, Székely A et al (2013) Reducing mortality in acute kidney injury patients: systematic review and international web-based survey. J Cardiothorac Vasc Anesth 27(6):1384–1398
11. Guyatt G, Gutterman D, Baumann MH et al (2006) Grading strength of recommendations and quality of evidence in clinical guidelines: report from an american college of chest physicians task force. Chest 129(1):174–181
12. Brienza N, Giglio MT, Marucci M, Fiore T (2009) Does perioperative hemodynamic optimization protect renal function in surgical patients? A meta-analytic study. Crit Care Med 37(6):2079–2090
13. Payen D, de Pont AC, Sakr Y et al (2008) A positive fluid balance is associated with a worse outcome in patients with acute renal failure. Crit Care 12(3):R74
14. Bouchard J, Soroko SB, Chertow GM et al (2009) Fluid accumulation, survival and recovery of kidney function in critically ill patients with acute kidney injury. Kidney Int 76(4):422–427
15. Sort P, Navasa M, Arroyo V et al (1999) Effect of intravenous albumin on renal impairment and mortality in patients with cirrhosis and spontaneous bacterial peritonitis. N Engl J Med 341(6):403–409
16. Wiedermann CJ, Dunzendorfer S, Gaioni LU et al (2010) Hyperoncotic colloids and acute kidney injury: a meta-analysis of randomized trials. Crit Care 14(5):R191
17. Brunkhorst FM, Engel C, Bloos F et al (2008) Intensive insulin therapy and pentastarch resuscitation in severe sepsis. N Engl J Med 358(2):125–139
18. Solanki P, Chawla A, Garg R et al (2003) Beneficial effects of terlipressin in hepatorenal syndrome: a prospective, randomized placebo-controlled clinical trial. J Gastroenterol Hepatol 18(2):152–156
19. Mehta RL, Pascual MT, Soroko S, Chertow GM, PICARD Study Group (2002) Diuretics, mortality, and nonrecovery of renal function in acute renal failure. JAMA 288(20):2547–2553
20. Keane WF, Hirata-Dulas CA, Bullock ML et al (1991) Adjunctive therapy with intravenous human immunoglobulin G improves survival of patients with acute renal failure. J Am Soc Nephrol 2(4):841–847
21. Marenzi G, Marana I, Lauri G et al (2003) The prevention of radiocontrast-agent-induced nephropathy by hemofiltration. N Engl J Med 349(14):1333–1340
22. Landoni G, Biondi-Zoccai GGL, Tumlin JA et al (2007) Beneficial impact of fenoldopam in critically ill patients with or at risk for acute renal failure: a meta-analysis of randomized clinical trials. Am J Kidney Dis 49(1):56–68
23. Zucchelli P, Pasquali S, Cagnoli L, Ferrari G (1988) Controlled plasma exchange trial in acute renal failure due to multiple myeloma. Kidney Int 33(6):1175–1180
24. Schiffl H, Lang SM, Fischer R (2002) Daily hemodialysis and the outcome of acute renal failure. N Engl J Med 346(5):305–310
25. Saudan P, Niederberger M, De Seigneux S et al (2006) Adding a dialysis dose to continuous hemofiltration increases survival in patients with acute renal failure. Kidney Int 70(7):1312–1317
26. Ronco C, Bellomo R, Homel P et al (2000) Effects of different doses in continuous veno-venous haemofiltration on outcomes of acute renal failure: a prospective randomised trial. Lancet 356(9223):26–30

27. Chung KK, Lundy JB, Matson JR et al (2009) Continuous venovenous hemofiltration in severely burned patients with acute kidney injury: a cohort study. Crit Care 13(3):R62
28. Kiser TH, Fish DN, Obritsch MD et al (2005) Vasopressin, not octreotide, may be beneficial in the treatment of hepatorenal syndrome: a retrospective study. Nephrol Dial Transplant 20(9):1813–1820
29. Gordon AC, Russell JA, Walley KR et al (2010) The effects of vasopressin on acute kidney injury in septic shock. Intensive Care Med 36(1):83–91
30. Kunt AT, Akgün S, Atalan N et al (2009) Furosemide infusion prevents the requirement of renal replacement therapy after cardiac surgery. Anadolu Kardiyol Derg 9(6):499–504
31. Oudemans-van Straaten HM, Bosman RJ, Koopmans M et al (2009) Citrate anticoagulation for continuous venovenous hemofiltration. Crit Care Med 37(2):545–552
32. Marenzi G, Assanelli E, Marana I et al (2006) N-acetylcysteine and contrast-induced nephropathy in primary angioplasty. N Engl J Med 354(26):2773–2782
33. Wijeysundera DN, Beattie WS, Rao V et al (2007) N-acetylcysteine for preventing acute kidney injury in cardiac surgery patients with pre-existing moderate renal insufficiency. Can J Anaesth 54(11):872–881
34. Bellomo R, Mansfield D, Rumble S et al (1993) A comparison of conventional dialytic therapy and acute continuous hemodiafiltration in the management of acute renal failure in the critically ill. Ren Fail 15(5):595–602
35. Seabra VF, Balk EM, Liangos O et al (2008) Timing of renal replacement therapy initiation in acute renal failure: a meta-analysis. Am J Kidney Dis 52(2):272–284
36. Demirkiliç U, Kuralay E, Yenicesu M et al (2004) Timing of replacement therapy for acute renal failure after cardiac surgery. J Card Surg 19(1):17–20

Part II

Interventions That May Reduce Mortality

Continuous Renal Replacement Therapy Versus Intermittent Haemodialysis: Impact on Clinical Outcomes

4

Johan Mårtensson and Rinaldo Bellomo

4.1 General Principles

Renal replacement therapy (RRT) is required to maintain water and electrolyte homeostasis and to remove waste products in critically ill patients with severe acute kidney injury (AKI). Mortality is close to 60 % in such patients, and survivors carry a significant risk of progression to chronic kidney disease (CKD) and dialysis-dependent end-stage renal disease (ESRD) [1]. Recent international consensus statements concluded that continuous RRT (CRRT) instead of intermittent haemodialysis (IHD) should not be routinely used with the intention to improve survival in critically ill patients with AKI [2]. Yet, CRRT is an attractive technique, which offers superior cardiovascular stability during water and solute removal compared to IHD. This is an important difference between the two techniques since haemodynamic stability during CRRT has been linked to improved renal functional recovery in critically ill patients with severe AKI [3].

J. Mårtensson (✉)
Department of Intensive Care, Austin Hospital,
145 Studley Road, Heidelberg, VIC 3084, Australia

Section of Anaesthesia and Intensive Care Medicine, Department of Physiology and Pharmacology, Karolinska Institutet, Stockholm, Sweden
e-mail: Johan.MARTENSSON@austin.org.au

R. Bellomo
Department of Intensive Care, Austin Hospital,
145 Studley Road, Heidelberg, VIC 3084, Australia

Australian and New Zealand Intensive Care Research Centre (ANZIC-RC), Department of Epidemiology and Preventive Medicine, Monash University, Melbourne, VIC, Australia
e-mail: Rinaldo.BELLOMO@austin.org.au

© Springer International Publishing Switzerland 2016

G. Landoni et al. (eds.), *Reducing Mortality in Acute Kidney Injury*,
DOI 10.1007/978-3-319-33429-5_4

4.2 Main Evidence

Early observational studies suggested a survival benefit with CRRT as compared to IHD [4]. Since then, several randomised controlled trials (RCTs) have compared CRRT versus IHD in a total of more than 1,100 patients with severe AKI (Table 4.1) [5–10]. The first trial, published in 2001, showed improved survival in IHD-treated patients [5]. However, significantly lower illness severity in the IHD group biased the results. After adjusting for group imbalances, no association between RRT modality and mortality was found. Subsequent trials have all failed to demonstrate improved survival or, as secondary end point, short-term renal recovery (dialysis-free status at hospital discharge) with CRRT. Meta-analyses support these findings [3, 11].

To date, no RCT has explored the impact of intermittent versus continuous RRT on chronic dialysis dependence beyond 90 days. Results from large observational studies, however, suggest higher long-term risk of ESRD in critically ill patients receiving IHD instead of CRRT [12] (Fig. 4.1), an association that appears particularly pronounced in patients with pre-existing CKD or cardiac failure [13].

In a meta-analysis of 16 observational studies, the risk of ESRD was twice as high among ICU patients treated with IHD than among ICU patients treated with CRRT (pooled relative risk 1.99, 95 % confidence interval [CI] 1.53–2.59) [3]. In a more recent, retrospective cohort study, 2004 CRRT patients were matched to 2004 IHD patients to assess the impact of RRT modality on ESRD risk 90 days after ICU admission [13]. Matching was based on the presence of CKD, mechanical ventilation and the propensity of receiving CRRT. Compared with IHD, treatment with CRRT was associated with a 25 % reduced risk of ESRD (hazard ratio [HR] 0.75,

Table 4.1 Peer-reviewed randomised controlled trials comparing IHD and CRRT with mortality as primary outcome

Authors	Year	*N*	CRRT intensity	IHD intensity	Mortality	Renal recovery[a]
Mehta et al. [5]	2001	166	NR	NR	No difference[b]	No difference
Gasparovic et al. [6]	2003	104	18–35 mL/kg/h	NR	No difference	NR
Augustine et al. [7]	2004	80	NR	NR	No difference	No difference
Uehlinger et al. [8]	2005	125	25.9 mL/min[c]	24.8 mL/min[c]	No difference	No difference
Vinsonneau et al. [9]	2006	360	29 mL/kg/h	NR	No difference	No difference
Lins et al. [10]	2009	316	NR	NR	No difference	No difference

NR not reported
[a]Short-term renal recovery
[b]After adjusting for imbalances in group assignment
[c]Average daily small solute clearance

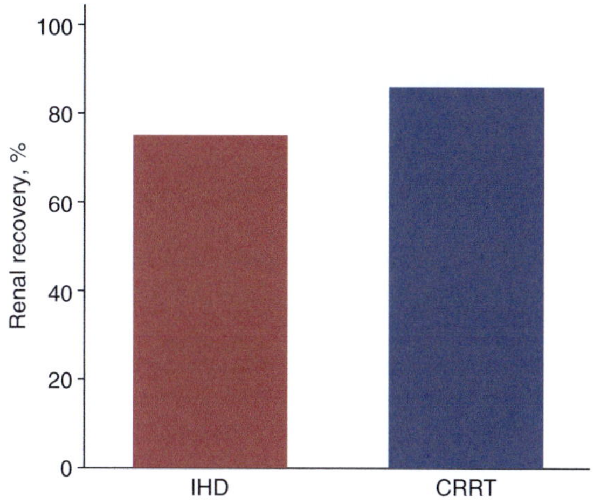

Fig. 4.1 Long-term renal recovery in critically ill patients treated with IHD or CRRT (Data from Schneider et al. [3] and Wald et al. [13])

95 % CI 0.65–0.87). The results of these studies strongly suggest that CRRT should be preferred over IHD during the early stages of critical illness.

4.3 Pathophysiological Principles

RRT has a major impact on cardiovascular stability. The degree of haemodynamic instability during RRT is a function of the intensity of solute and water removal and the rate of solute and water equilibrium between the vascular and interstitial compartments. When RRT starts, a large amount of osmotically active substances, such as urea, are removed from plasma water, which then becomes hypoosmotic relative to the interstitium. Consequently, an osmotic gradient is created allowing net water movement from the vascular into the interstitial compartment. Urea and other solutes will eventually, yet more slowly than water, move in the opposite direction to create equilibrium and vascular refilling of water from the interstitium.

IHD is a high-intensity treatment administered during short time intervals (usually 3 h three to four times/week). Several potential mechanisms related to treatment with IHD may be responsible for the observed long-term progression from acute to chronic kidney disease. Firstly, an instant drop in plasma urea concentration will occur during any IHD session. As a result, water movement to the relatively hyperosmotic interstitium will exceed vascular refilling and cause relative hypovolemia with an increased risk of hypotension, particularly in vasodilated patients and in patients with poor cardiac systolic function. Additionally, ultrafiltration of large fluid volumes (1–4 l) is usually required during each dialysis session to meet daily fluid intake and to avoid fluid overload. Such large-volume fluid removal contributes to hypovolemia and further increases the risk of hypotension. Even short episodes of hypotension increase the risk of progressive renal impairment in different populations [14, 15]. It is likely that IHD-induced hypotension contributes to persistent kidney damage that later progress to ESRD.

Secondly, the ability to maintain an even or negative daily fluid balance in haemodynamically unstable patients by intermittent fluid removal is limited by the operational characteristics of the IHD machine but, more importantly, by the patient's cardiovascular status. In fact, it was previously shown that RRT with IHD is associated with progressive fluid accumulation in critically ill patients [16]. Since severe organ oedema is a common trigger for starting RRT [17], further fluid gain will be poorly tolerated by such patients. In fact, a positive daily fluid balance during RRT was independently associated with prolonged need for RRT, increased ICU and hospital length of stay and increased mortality in a post hoc analysis of a large RCT [18].

Finally, plasma concentrations of important drugs such as antibiotics may be difficult to predict during IHD. Elevated plasma levels of nephrotoxic drugs between IHD sessions may contribute to kidney damage. In addition, sub-therapeutic antibiotic levels during IHD sessions may delay resolution of severe infections and recovery of associated organ failure.

In contrast to IHD, CRRT provides slow removal of water and waste products for up to 24 h per day. This prevents urea disequilibrium, allows simultaneous vascular refilling from the interstitium and thereby decreases the likelihood of hypotensive episodes. Moreover, antibiotic concentrations can more easily be maintained within therapeutic range.

4.4 Therapeutic Use

Solute removal during IHD is achieved by diffusion. Blood flow rates of 200–300 mL/min are typically delivered through a single-pass system. The countercurrent dialysate flow rates of 500–800 mL/min thereby markedly exceed blood flow rates. A further increase of the dialysate flow rate has minimal effect on solute clearance since the dialysate fluid does not become saturated during its passage through the filter. To achieve a higher dialysis dose, the blood flow rate needs to be increased. In addition, the pressure difference over the filter, the so-called transmembrane pressure, can be increased to achieve ultrafiltration and hence net fluid removal. Since IHD delivers high solute clearance over a relatively short time, it is therefore the preferential technique in early treatment of patients with life-threatening hyperkalaemia or severe intoxications with water-soluble substances. Moreover, IHD allows patient mobilisation between treatment sessions and may for that reason be the first choice in patients recovering from their critical illness.

Yet, IHD has potential drawbacks in the ICU setting. Firstly, the need for qualified dialysis staff may delay treatment. This is important since delayed RRT initiation in relation to accumulation of uremic toxins [19] or fluid [20] may adversely affect outcomes. Secondly, as discussed above, repeated hypotensive episodes during IHD are a likely risk factor for long-term CKD.

Finally, IHD can induce dialysis disequilibrium syndrome (DDS) characterised by cerebral oedema and seizures [21]. DDS is caused by rapid removal of urea (and other osmotically active substances) from the circulation, which creates an osmotic

Clinical Summary

Technique	Indications	Cautions	Side effects	Dose	Notes
IHD	1. ESRD 2. Severe AKI 3. Intoxications	Critically ill patients requiring cardiovascular support Raised intracranial pressure	Hypotension Seizures in patients with raised intracranial pressure	*Kt/V* 3.9/week[a,b]	May be preferred in patients undergoing frequent daily procedures or investigations or in mobilised patients
CRRT	1. Severe AKI 2. Intoxications	Difficult to achieve prescribed dose if frequent interruptions	Hypophosphatemia	20–25 mL/kg/h[b]	First choice in haemodynamically unstable patients and in patients with raised intracranial pressure

[a]Urea clearance (K) × dialysis time (t)/volume of urea distribution (V)

[b]Recommendations from kidney disease: Improving Global Outcomes 2012 guidelines [23]

gradient between brain and plasma. This gradient promotes water transport into the brain resulting in cerebral oedema [22]. IHD is therefore contraindicated in patients with head injury due to the risk of life-threatening increases in intracranial pressure in these patients.

Solute removal during CRRT can be achieved by convection (continuous venovenous haemofiltration (CVVH)), by diffusion (continuous venovenous haemodialysis (CVVHD)) or by a combination of both convection and diffusion (continuous venovenous haemodiafiltration (CVVHDF)). Replacement fluid is delivered pre- and/or post filter to maintain fluid balance during CVVH. Convective solute clearance is dictated by the ultrafiltration rate. Blood flow rates of 150–200 mL/min are typically used during CRRT and, unlike IHD, exceed dialysate flow rates (15–30 mL/min) during CVVHD and CVVHDF. Consequently, since the dialysate solution becomes saturated before it exits the filter, its flow rate needs to be increased in order to achieve higher diffusive clearance. Gentle fluid and solute removal during CRRT offer better cardiovascular stability and reduces the risk of DDS significantly. CRRT should therefore be considered the treatment of choice in haemodynamically unstable AKI patients and in AKI patients with increased or labile intracranial pressure.

Conclusions

Randomised controlled trials have failed to demonstrate survival benefit with CRRT compared to IHD in critically ill patients with AKI. The two techniques have, however, different advantages at different stages during the course of critical illness. Gentle water and solute removal during CRRT offer superior cardiovascular stability and should be preferred during the acute phase to minimise the risk of hypotensive episodes, which may contribute to long-term progression to CKD and ESRD. In contrast, IHD may be chosen to facilitate mobilisation during the recovery phase.

References

1. Gallagher M, Cass A, Bellomo R et al (2014) Long-term survival and dialysis dependency following acute kidney injury in intensive care: extended follow-up of a randomized controlled trial. PLoS Med 11(2), e1001601
2. Landoni G, Bove T, Szekely A et al (2013) Reducing mortality in acute kidney injury patients: systematic review and international web-based survey. J Cardiothorac Vasc Anesth 27(6):1384–1398
3. Schneider AG, Bellomo R, Bagshaw SM et al (2013) Choice of renal replacement therapy modality and dialysis dependence after acute kidney injury: a systematic review and meta-analysis. Intensive Care Med 39(6):987–997
4. Bellomo R, Mansfield D, Rumble S et al (1993) A comparison of conventional dialytic therapy and acute continuous hemodiafiltration in the management of acute renal failure in the critically ill. Ren Fail 15(5):595–602
5. Mehta RL, McDonald B, Gabbai FB et al (2001) A randomized clinical trial of continuous versus intermittent dialysis for acute renal failure. Kidney Int 60(3):1154–1163

6. Gasparovic V, Filipovic-Grcic I, Merkler M et al (2003) Continuous renal replacement therapy (CRRT) or intermittent hemodialysis (IHD) – what is the procedure of choice in critically ill patients? Ren Fail 25(5):855–862
7. Augustine JJ, Sandy D, Seifert TH et al (2004) A randomized controlled trial comparing intermittent with continuous dialysis in patients with ARF. Am J Kidney Dis 44(6):1000–1007
8. Uehlinger DE, Jakob SM, Ferrari P et al (2005) Comparison of continuous and intermittent renal replacement therapy for acute renal failure. Nephrol Dial Transplant 20(8):1630–1637
9. Vinsonneau C, Camus C, Combes A et al (2006) Continuous venovenous haemodiafiltration versus intermittent haemodialysis for acute renal failure in patients with multiple-organ dysfunction syndrome: a multicentre randomised trial. Lancet 368(9533):379–385
10. Lins RL, Elseviers MM, Van der Niepen P et al (2009) Intermittent versus continuous renal replacement therapy for acute kidney injury patients admitted to the intensive care unit: results of a randomized clinical trial. Nephrol Dial Transplant 24(2):512–518
11. Rabindranath K, Adams J, Macleod AM et al (2007) Intermittent versus continuous renal replacement therapy for acute renal failure in adults. Cochrane Database Syst Rev (3):CD003773
12. Rimes-Stigare C, Awad A, Martensson J et al (2012) Long-term outcome after acute renal replacement therapy: a narrative review. Acta Anaesthesiol Scand 56(2):138–146
13. Wald R, Shariff SZ, Adhikari NK et al (2014) The association between renal replacement therapy modality and long-term outcomes among critically ill adults with acute kidney injury: a retrospective cohort study. Crit Care Med 42(4):868–877
14. Walsh M, Devereaux PJ, Garg AX et al (2013) Relationship between intraoperative mean arterial pressure and clinical outcomes after noncardiac surgery: toward an empirical definition of hypotension. Anesthesiology 119(3):507–515
15. Asfar P, Meziani F, Hamel JF et al (2014) High versus low blood-pressure target in patients with septic shock. N Engl J Med 370(17):1583–1593
16. Bouchard J, Soroko SB, Chertow GM et al (2009) Fluid accumulation, survival and recovery of kidney function in critically ill patients with acute kidney injury. Kidney Int 76(4):422–427
17. Bellomo R, Cass A, Cole L et al (2009) Intensity of continuous renal-replacement therapy in critically ill patients. N Engl J Med 361(17):1627–1638
18. Bellomo R, Cass A, Cole L et al (2012) An observational study fluid balance and patient outcomes in the randomized evaluation of normal vs. augmented level of replacement therapy trial. Crit Care Med 40(6):1753–1760
19. Vaara ST, Reinikainen M, Wald R et al (2014) Timing of RRT based on the presence of conventional indications. Clin J Am Soc Nephrol 9(9):1577–1585
20. Vaara ST, Korhonen AM, Kaukonen KM et al (2012) Fluid overload is associated with an increased risk for 90-day mortality in critically ill patients with renal replacement therapy: data from the prospective FINNAKI study. Crit Care 16(5):R197
21. La Greca G, Biasioli S, Chiaramonte S et al (1982) Studies on brain density in hemodialysis and peritoneal dialysis. Nephron 31(2):146–150
22. Patel N, Dalal P, Panesar M (2008) Dialysis disequilibrium syndrome: a narrative review. Semin Dial 21(5):493–498
23. Lameire N, Kellum JA (2013) Contrast-induced acute kidney injury and renal support for acute kidney injury: a KDIGO summary (Part 2). Crit Care 17:205

May an "Early" Renal Replacement Therapy Improve Survival?

5

Giacomo Monti, Massimiliano Greco, and Luca Cabrini

5.1 General Principles

Renal replacement therapy (RRT) is the main supportive treatment for acute kidney injury (AKI). Traditionally, RRT has been primarily aimed at avoiding the life-threatening imbalances associated with kidney failure (metabolic acidosis, hyperkalemia, uremia, and/or fluid overload). More recently, researchers and clinicians have developed a different approach, often referred as "renal support," in which the underlying hypothesis is that earlier initiation of RRT may attenuate kidney damage as well as extrarenal organ injury.

However, even if a large meta-analysis suggested that "early RRT" could offer some survival benefits [1], there is no consensus for the optimal timing to start RRT in the setting of AKI in patients with critical illness due to different causes. This is primarily due to the lack of any widely agreed parameter, marker, or criteria to be used as a trigger to start RRT. Moreover, the definitions of "early" and "late" RRT vary largely even among studies where a similar trigger is chosen. Finally, the impact of timing of RRT initiation on outcome is difficult to assess: first, many studies have confounders, such as the use of diuretics, the inclusion of only septic patients, and the inclusion of mixed patients from a critically ill population and second, RRT is one name for many techniques changing in modality, dialyzer membrane, level of intensity, and frequency of application.

G. Monti, MD (✉) • M. Greco, MD • L. Cabrini, MD
IRCCS Ospedale San Raffaele, Università Vita-Salute San Raffaele,
Via Olgettina 60, Milan 20132, Italy
e-mail: monti.giacomo@hsr.it; greco.massimiliano@hsr.it; cabrini.luca@hsr.it

© Springer International Publishing Switzerland 2016

G. Landoni et al. (eds.), *Reducing Mortality in Acute Kidney Injury*,
DOI 10.1007/978-3-319-33429-5_5

5.2 Main Evidence

Evidence in this setting comes especially from observational studies, from a few randomized studies, and from two recent and large meta-analyses.

The meta-analysis by Seabra et al. [1] provides the most comprehensive insight about the impact of RRT timing on survival. It included 23 studies on intermittent hemodialysis (IHD) or continuous venovenous hemodiafiltration (CVVHDF) using a variety of dialyser types. Only four studies were randomized and one was quasi-randomized, overall including 270 patients. Sixteen were retrospective cohort studies, including the majority of patients (1832). Other 294 patients were included from mixed studies.

A range of different definitions of "early" and "late" RRT was used in the studies analyzed, related to both the level of a renal blood marker (usually urea but also creatinine) or the degree of clinical deterioration (e.g., urine output). Outcomes included mortality and recovery of renal function.

Generally speaking, the application of an "earlier" RRT has developed over the years. Indeed, when considering only the uremia level in the "late RRT" groups of the studies included in the meta-analysis (namely, the most restrictive approach to RRT initiation), and plotting it over the years of publication of the papers, a trend in reduction of the blood urea level which defines "late RRT" can be clearly seen (Fig. 5.1).

The primary analysis, which included the randomized and quasi-randomized studies, failed to show a statistically significant difference in mortality. However, a trend toward a reduced mortality was found. In fact, mortality was 66 % (25–80) in

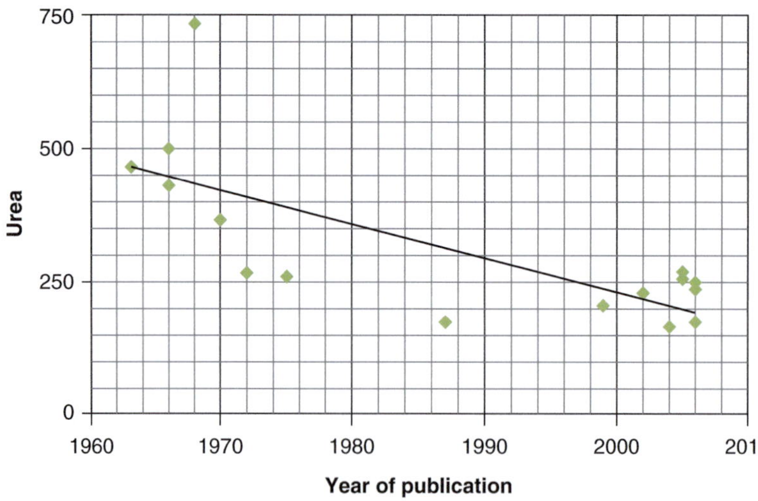

Fig. 5.1 The trend over years of the definition of "late RRT" in published studies (Data from Seabra et al. [1]). The graph shows a clear trend toward reduction. Urea (mg/dL) is expressed as blood urea nitrogen (BUN) × 2.14

the late RRT group, while early RRT was associated with a 36 % mortality risk reduction (relative risk [RR] 0.64, 95 % confidence interval [CI] 0.40–1.05, $p=0.08$). In detail, these 270 patients come from five studies, performed from 1975 to 2006. None of the studies used the same trigger criteria, two studies [2, 3] used intermittent hemodiafiltration, and two studies [4, 5] used continuous venovenous hemofiltration. In spite of considerable differences, these studies did not have significantly heterogeneous results.

Including in the meta-analysis data from the other 2,108 nonrandomized patients, the overall mortality rate was 68 % in the late RRT group, while it was significantly reduced (by 28 %) in the early RRT group (RR 0.72, 95 % CI 0.64–0.82, $p<0.001$).

Seabra and colleagues [1] also examined the possibility that early RRT could have an impact on recovery of renal failure, but no significant conclusion could be drawn.

At the time of the first international web-enabled consensus conference on mortality reduction in patients with or at risk for AKI [6], the meta-analysis by Seabra et al. [1] was the only evidence, together with a small retrospective cohort study with important methodological flaws [7], which was also included in the meta-analysis, suggesting that early institution of RRT might have a beneficial effect on survival in patients with AKI. However, according to the authors' conclusion, these results strongly encouraged to perform larger and adequately designed trials on the topic. Unfortunately, based on the data of the meta-analysis a study of adequate power should include over 1,000 patients.

A more recent meta-analysis [8] considered some of the papers included by Seabra and colleagues [1] but intentionally excluded older studies (i.e., those published before 1985) due to the considerable advances in available technology for providing RRT, the marked demographic transition of critically ill populations, and the evolution, generally speaking, of the interventions and technology available to support the critically ill. Overall 28-day mortality across the 15 trials included was 53.3 %. Early RRT initiation was associated with a reduced mortality as compared with late initiation (pooled odds ratio [OR] 0.45, 95 % CI 0.28–0.72, $p<0.001$). However, there was significant statistical heterogeneity (I^2 78 %, Q 63.7), most likely explained by differences in study design, particularly regarding operational definitions for RRT timing, and by the inability to account for heterogeneity in clinical practice patterns.

A small randomized study including 53 intensive care unit (ICU) patients affected by acute respiratory distress syndrome (ARDS), mostly caused by sepsis, was published in 2015 [9]. Patients were randomized to receive either early (less than 12 h from ICU admission) or late (more than 48 h) continuous RRT. Length of mechanical ventilation, oxygenation, survival, and some markers of inflammation were assessed. The authors found an overall beneficial effect of early RRT: shorter duration of mechanical ventilation (10 vs. 13 days, $p=0.0123$), higher PaO_2/FiO_2 ratio (220 vs. 178 mmHg, $p<0.05$), and a trend toward increased survival (22 % vs. 35 %, $p=0.32$). Moreover, early RRT was found to be potentially associated with removal of lung water and inflammatory cytokine TGF-β1 from both serum and bronchoalveolar lavage fluid.

Finally, an interesting retrospective observational study was conducted in Taiwan on 648 adult patients with postoperative AKI [10]. Patients were categorized according to the time between ICU admission and RRT initiation as the early (≤1 day), intermediate (2–3 days), and late (≥4 days) groups. Both the estimated probability of death and in-hospital mortality rates of the three groups represented U-shaped curves, with higher in-hospital mortality for both early and late groups compared to the intermediate one (59 %, 67 %, and 48 %, respectively, log rank $p=0.005$). It is noteworthy that, despite this quite big population included only postoperative patients, the causes of AKI were very variable, including sepsis, low cardiac output syndrome, and acute respiratory failure with extracorporeal membrane oxygenation (ECMO) support.

5.3 Pathophysiological Principles

When evaluating the timing of RRT and the potential benefits of an early treatment, the cause of AKI should be considered. In ICU patients, AKI is usually secondary to nonrenal diseases or conditions, whereas primary kidney diseases are not frequent in this specific setting [11]. Generally speaking, if RRT could help to treat the primary disease, probably an early RRT could be more useful than a late one. As an example, if AKI is caused by low cardiac output syndrome due to a massive acute myocardial infarction (AMI), early RRT will not contribute to reversal of AMI and, thereafter, will probably not enhance survival as compared with a late approach.

On the contrary, it could be expected that an early RRT approach can provide enhanced survival and a reduction in kidney failure in patients with sepsis since cytokines and other inflammatory mediators are involved in the pathogenesis of both shock and AKI in septic patients, and RRT allows removal of these mediators.

Nevertheless, the pathophysiology of sepsis-associated AKI is complex and multifactorial and includes intrarenal hemodynamic changes, endothelial dysfunction, intraglomerular thrombosis, infiltration of inflammatory cells in the renal parenchyma, and tubular obstruction by necrotic cells and debris. Evidence now suggests that the immune responses induced by sepsis involve the activation, in a sequential manner, of both pro- and anti-inflammatory mechanisms [12].

Although RRT should remove inflammatory cytokines and partly modulates plasma cytokines, outcomes in septic patients do not appear to be affected by RRT, regardless of the dose applied [13]. This may be due to the timing of RRT implementation and to patient selection but also to the limited effectiveness of standard filtration/dialysis membranes in removing cytokines, most of which are soluble in water and have a midrange molecular weight. This limited effectiveness is most probably due to the limited pore size of standard membranes for blood purification [13].

Maybe, if an immunoregulatory effect of RRT exists, the therapeutic window where RRT can be useful is early in the history of the disease, and thereafter an early approach could be more effective. Moreover, to cope with the mechanical issues in cytokine removal, different techniques have been developed. Coupled plasma filtration and adsorption (CPFA) separates plasma from blood by means of a plasma filter. After, plasma passes through a synthetic resin cartridge for adsorption and is returned to the blood. Adsorption is very effective in removing large molecules. Direct blood hemoperfusion with resins such as polymyxin B may be also performed. However, the effectiveness of these techniques has not yet been adequately evaluated [14].

Another setting where early RRT could be beneficial, in terms of survival, is respiratory failure. It has been shown that a restrictive strategy of fluid administration increases survival in ARDS patients [15]. On the contrary, especially in patients with sepsis-associated ARDS, a fluid overload is often present because of the need for large volumes of fluids in order to achieve hemodynamic stability. In ARDS, ventilatory treatment generally requires high positive intrathoracic pressure that may reduce cardiac output and cause water and sodium retention and, accordingly, reduced urine production. Moreover, biotrauma caused by mechanical ventilation, especially with tidal volumes over 6 mL/kg, leads to the systemic release of proinflammatory cytokines that can cause renal failure [16]. Thus, fluid overload and physiological stimuli to fluid retention, inflammation, and low renal blood flow often coexist in ARDS [13]. RRT may potentially revert all these conditions, and some specific studies already exist [9]. As for sepsis, some in-series techniques have been developed which can remove carbon dioxide from blood and allow a further reduction in tidal volumes. However, the possible survival benefits are still to be investigated [17].

5.4 Clinical Considerations

If early start of RRT seems to be not strongly associated with survival benefits, avoiding or delaying RRT is associated with higher mortality and increased hospital and ICU length of stay [13]. Accordingly, when a clinician has to decide "when" to start RRT, the balance between risks and benefits should be addressed, and complications of RRT should be considered. The cost of early RRT is, other than the economical one, the possibility of developing complications from a treatment that may not be strictly necessary. Probably, the only specific complication of an early approach comes from the loss of amino acids, catecholamines, and other compounds caused by RRT. In particular, drug dosing during RRT can be difficult and, mainly in septic patients, adjusting dosage and frequency of administration of antibiotics must be considered. Indeed, it has been shown that it could be difficult to achieve adequate blood levels of antibiotics during RRT [18]. When RRT is started early, it could be even more difficult to achieve a sufficient concentration of antibiotics, especially in the early phase of sepsis, where also other factors can lead to low antibiotic level (change in volume of distribution, low albumin levels, fluid challenges [19]).

Timing of treatment should not be considered in isolation but along with the treatment dose used, from which depends, in turn, the time needed to achieve uremic waste products control [20]. When RRT is started early, the concentration of wasting products will be lower and probably a low-intensity technique with the prescription of low dose will be adequate.

A widely agreed definition of "early" RRT is still missing. The most commonly accepted criteria to start RRT in acute care settings, as reported by Bellomo et al. [21], are summarized in Table 5.1. As suggested by Gibney et al. [22], an "early" approach to RRT could be defined in many ways:

- According to a surrogate biochemical marker, such as blood urea nitrogen (BUN), an "early" trigger value may be set at 38 mg/dL and a "late" value at 60 mg/dL (mean value of published studies).
- According to the onset time of oliguria, a urine output less than 30 mL/h for 3 h may be an indication to an "early" approach.
- According to the time from ICU admission.
- According to the level of fluid overload.

However, a clear and validated definition of "early" and "late" is still missing for most of these criteria.

Regard to the underlying condition which causes AKI, sepsis and ARDS are probably the two most promising clinical settings in which an early approach to RRT could be more beneficial in terms of survival. Moreover, as mentioned, specific extracorporeal techniques can be coupled to RRT in these settings in order to enhance its capabilities.

As stated by Landoni et al. [6], only a weak recommendation can be made, at present, for an "early" use of RRT. Large and adequately designed randomized clinical trial are certainly needed on this topic. Hopefully, new insights about timing of RRT may be provided by two investigations which are currently on the way.

The first one will enroll patients with RIFLE "F" (failure) AKI (threefold increase in serum creatinine as compared to baseline, an absolute creatinine value ≥4.0 mg/dL (354 μmol/L), a urine output ≤0.3 mL kg^{-1} h^{-1} for ≥24 h, or anuria for ≥12 h), defining an early approach to RRT as a maximum delay for RRT start of 12 h and a late approach as RRT beginning after 48 h from diagnosis of AKI [23].

Table 5.1 Current conventional indications for RRT initiation

Criteria
Anuria for 6 h
Severe oliguria (<200 mL over 12 h)
Hyperkalemia (>6.6 mmol/L)
Severe metabolic acidosis (pH<7.2 despite normal or low pCO_2)
Volume overload (especially unresponsive to diuretics)
Pronounced azotemia (urea >30 mmol/L or creatinine >300 μmol/L)
Clinical complications of uremia

Adapted with permission from Bellomo et al. [21]

The second ongoing study will enroll critically ill patients receiving intravenous catecholamines or invasive mechanical ventilation and presenting with KDIGO classification stage 3 AKI (see Chap. 2). In the "early" strategy, RRT is initiated immediately. In the "delayed" strategy, the clinical conditions and the metabolic status are strictly monitored, and RRT is initiated only when one or more of the following criteria of severity occur: oliguria or anuria for more than 72 h, serum urea concentration >40 mmol/L, serum potassium concentration >6 mmol/L, serum potassium concentration >5.5 mmol/L persisting despite medical treatment, arterial blood pH <7.15, and acute pulmonary edema with severe hypoxemia unresponsive to diuretic therapy [24].

Clinical Summary

Technique	Indications	Cautions	Side effects	Notes
Early RRT	"Classical" indications to RRT, positive fluid balance, acute respiratory distress syndrome, severe sepsis	Survival benefit not clearly demonstrated	Metabolic (lost of amino acids, catecholamines, and other compounds) Possible difficulties in drugs dosing requiring dose adjusting Vascular access side effects Anticoagulation side effects	A widely agreed definition of "early" RRT is still missing

References

1. Seabra VF, Balk EF, Liangos E et al (2008) Timing of renal replacement therapy initiation in acute renal failure: a meta-analysis. Am J Kidney Dis 52:272–284
2. Conger JD (1975) A controlled evaluation of prophylactic dialysis in post-traumatic acute renal failure. J Trauma 15:1056–1063
3. Durmaz I, Yagdi T, Calkavur T et al (2003) Prophylactic dialysis in patients with renal dysfunction undergoing on-pump coronary artery bypass surgery. Ann Thorac Surg 75:859–864
4. Bouman CSC, Oudemans-Van Straaten HM, Tijssen JGP et al (2002) Effects of early high-volume continuous venovenous hemofiltration on survival and recovery of renal function in intensive care patients with acute renal failure: a prospective, randomized trial. Crit Care Med 30:2205–2211
5. Koo JR, Yoon JW, Oh JE et al (2006) Prospective evaluation of early continuous venovenous hemofiltration on the outcome in patients with severe sepsis or septic shock. J Am Soc Nephrol 17:50A (abstract)
6. Landoni G, Bove T, Székely A et al (2013) Reducing mortality in acute kidney injury patients: systematic review and international web-based survey. J Cardiothorac Vasc Anesth 27:1384–1398
7. Demirkiliç U, Kuralay E, Yenicesu M et al (2004) Timing of replacement therapy for acute renal failure after cardiac surgery. J Card Surg 19:17–20

8. Karvellas CJ, Farhat MR, Sajjad I et al (2011) A comparison of early versus late initiation of renal replacement therapy in critically ill patients with acute kidney injury: a systematic review and meta-analysis. Crit Care 15:R72
9. Han F, Sun R, Ni Y et al (2015) Early initiation of continuous renal replacement therapy improves clinical outcomes in patients with acute respiratory distress syndrome. Am J Med Sci 349:199–205
10. Shiao CC, Ko KJ, Wu VC et al (2012) U-curve association between timing of renal replacement therapy initiation and in-hospital mortality in postoperative acute kidney injury. PLoS ONE 7, e42952
11. Uchino S, Kellum JA, Bellomo R et al (2005) Acute renal failure in critically ill patients: a multinational, multicenter study. JAMA 294:813–818
12. Zarjou A, Agarwal A (2011) Sepsis and acute kidney injury. J Am Soc Nephrol 22:999–1006
13. Ronco C, Ricci Z, De Backer D et al (2015) Renal replacement therapy in acute kidney injury: controversy and consensus. Crit Care 19:146
14. Klein DJ, Foster D, Schorr CA et al (2014) The EUPHRATES trial (evaluating the use of polymyxin B hemoperfusion in a randomized controlled trial of adults treated for endotoxemia and septic shock): study protocol for a randomized controlled trial. Trials 15:218
15. National Heart, Lung, and Blood Institute Acute Respiratory Distress Syndrome (ARDS) Clinical Trials Network, Wiedemann HP, Wheeler AP, Bernard GR et al (2006) Comparison of two fluid-management strategies in acute lung injury. New Engl J Med 354:2564–2575
16. Jerng JS, Hsu YC, Wu HD et al (2007) Role of the renin-angiotensin system in ventilator-induced lung injury: an in vivo study in a rat model. Thorax 62:527–535
17. Terragni P, Maiolo G, Ranieri VM (2012) Role and potentials of low-flow CO(2) removal system in mechanical ventilation. Curr Opin Crit Care 18:93–98
18. Roberts DM, Roberts JA, Roberts MS et al (2012) Variability of antibiotic concentrations in critically ill patients receiving continuous renal replacement therapy: a multicentre pharmacokinetic study. Crit Care Med 40:1523–1528
19. Gonçalves-Pereira J, Póvoa P (2011) Antibiotics in critically ill patients: a systematic review of the pharmacokinetics of B-lactams. Crit Care 15:R206
20. Joannidis M, Forni LG (2011) Clinical review: timing of renal replacement therapy. Crit Care 15:223
21. Bellomo R, Kellum JA, Ronco C (2012) Acute kidney injury. Lancet 380:756–766
22. Gibney RT, Noel SM, Bagshaw DJ, Johnston C (2008) When should renal replacement therapy for acute kidney injury be initiated and discontinued? Blood Purif 26:473–484
23. Barbar SD, Binquet C, Monchi M et al (2014) Impact on mortality of the timing of renal replacement therapy in patients with severe acute kidney injury in septic shock: the IDEAL-ICU study (initiation of dialysis early versus delayed in the intensive care unit): study protocol for a randomized controlled trial. Trials 15:270
24. Gaudry S, Hajage D, Schortgen F et al (2015) Comparison of two strategies for initiating renal replacement therapy in the intensive care unit: study protocol for a randomized controlled trial (AKIKI). Trials 16:170

Increased Intensity of Renal Replacement Therapy to Reduce Mortality in Patients with Acute Kidney Injury

6

Zaccaria Ricci and Stefano Romagnoli

6.1 General Principles

Because initial studies showed a direct relationship between the intensity of renal replacement therapy (RRT) and survival, both for intermittent and continuous techniques [1–3], great attention has been paid to identify the optimal "dose" of RRT in the last 10 years.

Dose of RRT may be represented by the *efficiency* of the treatment, which can in turn be expressed as clearance (K) that is the amount of blood cleared of toxins and waste products by the extracorporeal circuit during a given period of time [4]. The concept of clearance needs to be referred to a particular solute. Urea is widely adopted as uremic toxin marker in clinical practice, and its clearance is most commonly used to quantify RRT efficiency and, accordingly, dose. Given that RRT is usually performed over several days or weeks, it is important to provide information about the total time during which the treatment clearance is delivered. The *intensity* of treatment (Fig. 6.1) is thus expressed as the product of clearance and the effective time (t) of treatment (Kt) [4]. Including the downtime (i.e., the amount of time in which the treatment is interrupted), a significant difference could be found between the prescribed and the actually delivered doses. Finally, considering the entire pool of solutes that needs to be cleared, the *efficacy* of treatment (Fig. 6.1) can be

Z. Ricci, MD (✉)
Pediatric Cardiac Intensive Care Unit, Department of Cardiology and Cardiac Surgery, Bambino Gesù Children's Hospital, IRCCS, Piazza S. Onofrio 4, Rome 00165, Italy
e-mail: z.ricci@libero.it

S. Romagnoli, MD
Section of Anesthesiology and Intensive Care, Department of Health Science, University of Florence, Florence, Italy

Department of Anesthesia and Intensive Care, Azienda Ospedaliero-Universitaria Careggi, Florence, Italy
e-mail: stefano-romagnoli@hotmail.com

© Springer International Publishing Switzerland 2016

G. Landoni et al. (eds.), *Reducing Mortality in Acute Kidney Injury*,
DOI 10.1007/978-3-319-33429-5_6

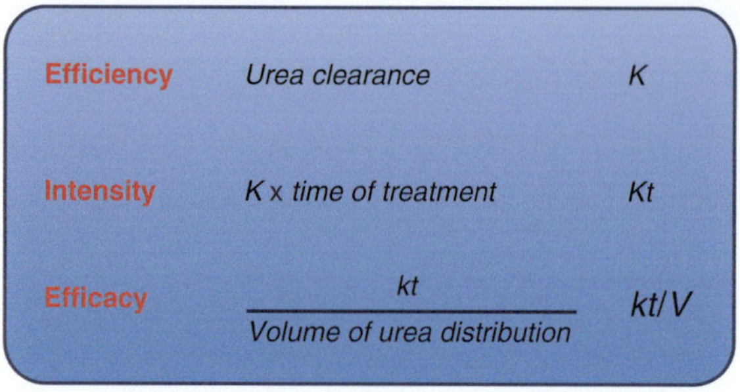

Fig. 6.1 Defining dose of renal replacement therapy (see text)

expressed as the ratio between the intensity and the volume of distribution (V) of the marker solute (*Kt*/*V*) [4]. Considering all these concepts during the prescription phase of RRT, it has seemed reasonable, since the birth of critical care nephrology [5], that an adequate treatment should have to be delivered to critically ill patients. In a few words, the idea was to provide "intense" blood purification, generally proportional to the severity of critical illness. However, back in the late 1980s, RRT machines used in the intensive care units (ICUs) were mostly adapted from the chronic hemodialysis ward, or in any case lacked several of current automatisms which are routinely applied to third- and fourth-generation RRT machines, and were probably unsuited for providing accurate and targeted treatments to critically ill patients with acute kidney injury (AKI) [6]. At that time, accordingly, RRT was certainly mostly underdosed. In this chapter, the available literature is analyzed with the aim to identify the current "optimal" dose of RRT in ICU patients with AKI, as well as to clarify whether and to what extent an increased treatment dose/intensity might provide a survival benefit in these patients.

6.2 Main Evidence

Several efforts have been made in the literature in order to define the most adequate RRT dose in AKI: the underlying idea is that RRT delivery may imply a dose-dependent range, where treatment efficiency correlates with outcomes, and a dose-independent range in which further dose increases will not result in additional benefits for the patients. Accordingly, during the last decade, the dose that was first shown to be associated to better patient outcome ($\geq$35 mL kg^{-1} h^{-1}) has been considered a milestone of critical care nephrology [1]. In particular, in 2000 Ronco et al. [1] randomized 425 ICU patients with acute renal failure (ARF) to receive continuous venovenous hemofiltration (CVVH) at 20, 35, or 45 mL kg^{-1} h^{-1} and found a significantly higher mortality in the 20 mL kg^{-1} h^{-1} group, as compared with the other two groups (which had similar survival rates). This study also suggested that post-dilution hemofiltration at higher does (45 mL kg^{-1} h^{-1}) may be indicated in specific conditions such as sepsis. The hypothesis that an increased intensity of RRT may improve survival was apparently confirmed also in patients receiving intermittent hemodialysis (IHD). In 2002, in fact, Schiffl et al. [2] randomized 160 ARF patients to either daily or conventional (i.e., on alternate days) IHD and showed a significant reduction in mortality in the daily dialysis group (28 % vs. 46 %, $p=0.01$). Interestingly, a few years later, Saudan et al. [3] evaluated the effect of additional RRT dose, delivered by adding a continuous diffusive technique to a purely convective treatment, in 206 ICU patients with ARF: again, patients receiving continuous venovenous hemodiafiltration (CVVHDF) showed a significant improvement in 90-day survival as compared with patients receiving CVVH (59 % vs. 34 %, $p=0.0005$).

More recently, however, two large multicenter randomized clinical trials examined the issue of the optimal RRT dose in ICU patients with AKI and the effect of increased intensity of RRT on mortality: the Randomized Evaluation of Normal versus Augmented Level of RRT (RENAL) study [7] and the Veterans Affairs/National institutes of Health Acute Renal Failure Trial Network (ATN) study [8].

In the RENAL trial [7], 1,508 patients were randomized to receive post-dilution CVVHDF with an effluent flow of either 25 or 40 mL kg^{-1} h^{-1}. The ATN study [8] included 1,124 patients who were randomly assigned to either 20 mL kg^{-1} h^{-1} CVVHDF or thrice-weekly IHD. Both studies failed to demonstrate that higher RRT doses were associated with better outcomes, except for a septic subgroup of the RENAL study with a reduced mortality when a higher dose was applied (odds ratio [OR] 0.84, 95 % confidence interval [CI] 0.62–1.12). However, under-dialysis should be always avoided in critically ill patients with AKI, and great attention should be paid in order to minimize the discrepancy between the prescribed and the actually delivered dose.

In light of this major issue, RRT downtime (defined as the overall time of RRT "standstill" over 24 h) was specifically explored in the "DOse REsponse Multicenter International collaborative initiative" (DO-RE-MI) [9]. Membrane clotting, vascular access issues (inducing physicians to modify the setting), and prescription errors (due to lack of knowledge) were the main contributors to continuous RRT (CRRT) stop. Therefore, if a "minimal" dose of 20–25 mL kg^{-1} h^{-1} (according to RENAL and ATN studies) should be prescribed, physicians should be advised to overprescribe the dose of at least 25 % (targeting 30–35 mL kg^{-1} h^{-1}), in order to limit the downtime effect.

Two important post hoc analyses of the RENAL trial were performed [10, 11]. The first suggested that fluid balance, rather than RRT dose, may actually affect patients' outcomes (see Chap. 19) [10]. In fact, the authors found that mean daily fluid balance among survivors was −234 mL/day compared with +560 mL/day among non-survivors ($p<0.0001$) and that a negative fluid balance was independently associated with favorable outcomes, including survival, RRT days, mechanical ventilation days, and both ICU and hospital length of stay. The second post hoc analysis examined acid-base balance and vasopressor utilization in the subgroup of patients with metabolic acidosis [11]. This study showed that the high-intensity group had a greater increase in mean arterial pressure from baseline to 24 h (7 ± 3 vs. 0 ± 3 mmHg, $p<0.01$) and a greater decrease in norepinephrine dose (from 12.5 to 3.5 vs. 5 to 2.5 μg/min, $p<0.05$). Despite a similar improvement in acid-base balance was observed in both groups, strong ion gap seemed to be better corrected by high-dose RRT. Although the authors acknowledged that a mechanistic analysis of the physiological effects induced by high-intensity RRT cannot be provided, they suggested that a more efficient removal of biologic mediators which are responsible for hypotension or vasodilation might be the potential mechanism of the observed hemodynamic improvement. Indeed, the changes in strong ion gap may indicate the removal of some of these mediators [11].

Finally, Uchino et al. [12] analyzed data from two multicenter investigations, the Beginning and Ending Supportive Therapy (BEST) study [13] and the Japanese Society for physician and trainees Intensive Care (JSEPTIC) trial [14], including 1,006 patients from 54 ICUs around the world and 343 patients from 12 Japanese ICUs, respectively. They found that AKI patients receiving low-dose CRRT (14.3 mL kg^{-1} h^{-1}) had not a worse short-term outcome as compared with patients receiving CRRT at doses closer to those currently considered as standard (20.4 mL kg^{-1} h^{-1}).

6.3 Pathophysiological Principles

One of the key issues of the modern concept of RRT is the clinical target: deriving from nephrology considerations, urea is the main solute that has been referred as the biomarker indicating how efficiently solutes are removed. However, urea is not the only solute which accumulates due to kidney injury and its kinetic of removal and volume of distribution differ by the other uremic toxins [15]. Considering urea as a target solute could result particularly useless in ICU patients. In fact, unlike patients with chronic kidney disease (CKD), uremic symptoms are rarely observed in the ICU, and they usually do not affect the clinical decision about CRRT in these patients. Other target solutes rather than urea should be considered in ICU patients. In particular, CRRT should be addressed to specific targets in specific clinical conditions (e.g., myoglobin in patients with compartment syndrome, interleukins during sepsis, novel biomarkers in case of early AKI, fluid balance in case of fluid overload). This concept would also redefine the concept of adequacy itself, which should probably include not only the amount of RRT to provide but also the exact circuits, filters, machines, and timing to be applied.

6.4 Therapeutic Use

A specific treatment that can be defined as "adequate" for all ICU patients in all conditions does not exist but, like mechanical ventilation, CRRT should be continuously tailored on patients' characteristics and their actual clinical needs.

Advantages and disadvantages of the different RRT modalities are summarized in Table 6.1 (see also Chap. 4).

Although three studies suggested a survival advantage with higher effluent dose [1], more frequent (daily) IHD [2], and the adjunct of continuous dialysis to CVVH [3], respectively, subsequent studies failed to confirm these findings.

Table 6.1 Advantages and disadvantages of different renal replacement therapy (RRT) modalities

RRT modality	Advantages	Disadvantages
Intermittent (IHD)	Rapid removal of toxins and circulating solutes Reduced downtime for diagnostic and therapeutic procedures Reduced exposure to anticoagulation Lower cost than CRRT	Rapid fluid removal and frequent hypotension Dialysis disequilibrium and risk of cerebral edema Technically complex
Prolonged (SLEDD)	Slower volume and solute removal than IHD Faster solutes clearance than CRRT Reduced downtime than CRRT Reduced exposure to anticoagulation than CRRT	Faster volume and solute removal than CRRT (increased risk for hypotension and disequilibrium syndrome in prone patients) Technically complex
Continuous (CRRT)	Continuous removal of toxins and solutes (avoid concentration rebound) Hemodynamic tolerability Easy control of fluid balance Avoid disequilibrium syndrome User-friendly machines	Slower solutes clearance than IHD Need for prolonged anticoagulation Reduced possibility of patient's mobilization Hypothermia Increased costs than IHD

IHD intermittent hemodialysis, *SLEDD* sustained low-efficiency daily dialysis, *CRRT* continuous RRT

Accordingly, an increase in RRT intensity in order to reduce mortality cannot be recommended [16].

Currently, a CRRT dose prescription below 20 mL kg^{-1} h^{-1} and over 35 mL kg^{-1} h^{-1} may be definitely identified as the dose-dependent range [17] (Fig. 6.2). In fact, reducing RRT intensity below 20 mL kg^{-1} h^{-1} is likely to negatively affect outcomes due to under-dialysis, while increasing it above 35 mL kg^{-1} h^{-1} might lead to electrolyte disorders and removal of nutrients and drugs, also potentially reducing survival. Conversely, prescriptions between 20 and 35 mL kg^{-1} h^{-1} can be considered as practice dependent: within this range, variables such as timing, patients' characteristics, comorbidities, or concomitant supportive pharmacological therapies may have a significant role in affecting patients' outcome and should trigger a careful prescription and a close monitoring of dose delivery.

Nowadays, a delivered dose (without downtime) between 20 and 25 mL kg^{-1} h^{-1} may be considered as clinically acceptable [17]. From a practical standpoint, considering that average downtime reduces delivered dose by 10–20 %, it might be recommended to prescribe 25–35 mL kg^{-1} h^{-1} in order to achieve an actual dose of at least 20–25 mL kg^{-1} h^{-1}. A dose prescription above 35 mL kg^{-1} h^{-1}, which is also associated to increased costs [18], is currently not recommended in any clinical condition.

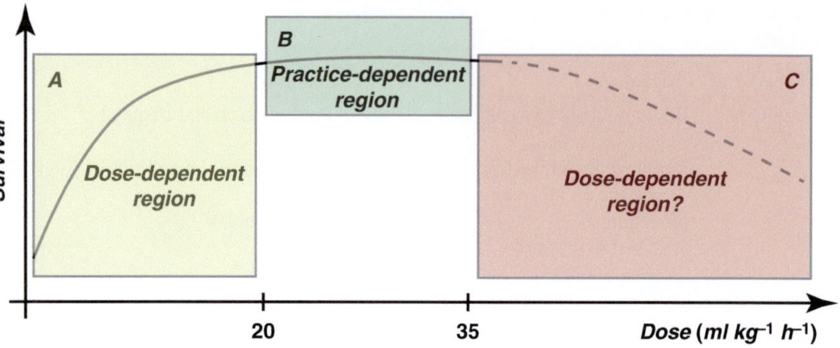

Fig. 6.2 Relationship between delivered dose and patient's survival. Below 20 mL kg^{-1} h^{-1} (panel **a**), the higher the dose the higher patients' survival (dose-dependent region). Above this limit, further increase in dose prescription (up to 35 mL kg^{-1} h^{-1}) may not influence patients' survival (panel **b**). In this range, other variables (e.g., time of treatment, optimization of blood perfusion, drug adjustments) may influence the outcome (practice-dependent region). With further increase of prescribed dose (over 35 mL kg^{-1} h^{-1}), electrolyte disorders and removal of nutrients and drugs (e.g., antibiotics) may occur, potentially reducing survival (panel **c**)

Clinical Summary

Strategy	Side effects	Dose	Notes
Increased intensity of renal replacement therapy	Possible electrolyte disorders and removal of nutrients and drugs (e.g., antibiotics) with effluent dose >35 mL kg^{-1} h^{-1} Increased costs	Increased intensity intended as: Increased effluent dose (≥35 mL kg^{-1} h^{-1}) Daily (rather than alternate-day) dialysis	None recommended in order to reduce mortality A targeted approach depending on the clinical condition may be rather advisable

References

1. Ronco C, Bellomo R, Homel P et al (2000) Effects of different doses in continuous venovenous hemofiltration on outcomes of acute renal failure: a prospective randomised trial. Lancet 356:26–30
2. Schiffl H, Lang SM, Fischer R (2002) Daily hemodialysis and the outcome of acute renal failure. N Engl J Med 346:305–310
3. Saudan P, Niederberger M, De Seigneux S et al (2006) Adding a dialysis dose to continuous hemofiltration increases survival in patients with acute renal failure. Kidney Int 70:1312–1317

4. Ricci Z, Bellomo R, Ronco C (2006) Dose of dialysis in acute renal failure. Clin J Am Soc Nephrol 1:380–388
5. Ronco C, Bellomo R, Feriani M et al (1998) Critical care nephrology: the time has come. Kidney Int Suppl 66:S1–S2
6. Ronco C, Ricci Z (2015) Pediatric continuous renal replacement: 20 years later. Intensive Care Med 41:985–993
7. RENAL Replacement Therapy Study Investigators, Bellomo R, Cass A, Cole L et al (2009) Intensity of continuous renal-replacement therapy in critically ill patients. N Engl J Med 361:1627–1638
8. VA/NIH Acute Renal Failure Trial Network, Palevsky PM, Zhang JH, O'Connor TZ et al (2008) Intensity of renal support in critically ill patients with acute kidney injury. N Engl J Med 359:7–20
9. Monti G, Herrera M, Kindgen-Milles D et al (2007) The DOse REsponse Multicentre International Collaborative Initiative (DO-RE-MI). Contrib Nephrol 156:434–443
10. RENAL Replacement Therapy Study Investigators, Bellomo R, Cass A, Cole L et al (2012) An observational study fluid balance and patient outcomes in the randomized evaluation of normal vs. augmented level of replacement therapy trial. Crit Care Med 40:1753–1760
11. Bellomo R, Lipcsey M, Calzavacca P et al (2013) Early acid-base and blood pressure effects of continuous renal replacement therapy intensity in patients with metabolic acidosis. Intensive Care Med 39:429–436
12. Uchino S, Toki N, Takeda K et al (2013) Validity of low-intensity continuous renal replacement therapy. Crit Care Med 41:2584–2591
13. Uchino S, Kellum J, Bellomo R et al (2005) Acute renal failure in critically ill patients: a multinational, multicenter study. JAMA 294:813–818
14. Yasuda H, Uchino S, Uji M, Japanese Society for Physicians and Trainees in Intensive Care Clinical Trial Group et al (2014) The lower limit of intensity to control uremia during continuous renal replacement therapy. Crit Care 18:539
15. Ricci Z, Romagnoli S, Ronco C (2011) Renal support. Minerva Anestesiol 77:1204–1215
16. Landoni G, Bove T, Székely A et al (2013) Reducing mortality in acute kidney injury patients: systematic review and international web-based survey. J Cardiothorac Vasc Anesth 27(6):1384–1398
17. Kidney Disease: Improving Global Outcomes (KDIGO) Acute Kidney Injury Work Group (2012) KDIGO clinical practice guideline for acute kidney injury. Kidney Int Suppl 2:1–138
18. Srisawat N, Lawsin L, Uchino S, BEST Kidney Investigators et al (2010) Cost of acute renal replacement therapy in the intensive care unit: results from The Beginning and Ending Supportive Therapy for the Kidney (BEST Kidney) study. Crit Care 14:R46

7 Citrate Anticoagulation to Reduce Mortality in Patients Needing Continuous Renal Replacement Therapy

Massimiliano Greco, Giacomo Monti, and Luca Cabrini

7.1 General Principles

Acute kidney injury (AKI) is an independent predictor of mortality in critically ill patients [1]. Continuous renal replacement therapy (CRRT) developed as a treatment for renal failure in patients who are unable to undergo standard dialytic treatment due to hemodynamic instability.

Several different renal replacement therapies are now available, including continuous or intermittent techniques. These strategies need some form of anticoagulation to increase circuit survival and to reduce the complications associated with circuit clotting such as thrombocytopenia. Continuous intravenous administration of unfractionated heparin (UH) is the most common approach. However, systemic anticoagulation with UH is associated with potentially serious adverse effects such as bleeding and heparin-induced thrombocytopenia (HIT) [2]. Regional anticoagulation with citrate has been proposed as an effective and safe mean for anticoagulation during CRRT. Recently, the first international web-based consensus conference on mortality reduction in patients with or at risk for AKI [3] included citrate anticoagulation for continuous venovenous hemofiltration (CVVH) among drugs and techniques which may increase survival in critically ill patients with AKI.

7.2 Main Evidence

Oudemans-van Straaten et al. [4] conducted a non-blinded randomized controlled trial to compare the effect of nadroparin, a low molecular weight heparin (LMWH), and citrate regional anticoagulation in critically ill patients on CVVH

M. Greco (✉) • G. Monti • L. Cabrini
Department of Anesthesia and Intensive Care, San Raffaele Scientific Institute, via Olgettina 60, Milan 20132, Italy
e-mail: greco.massimiliano@hsr.it; monti.giacomo@hsr.it; cabrini.luca@hsr.it

© Springer International Publishing Switzerland 2016

G. Landoni et al. (eds.), *Reducing Mortality in Acute Kidney Injury*,
DOI 10.1007/978-3-319-33429-5_7

from a single-center teaching hospital. A total of 215 patients were randomized. Adverse events, including bleeding complications, were more frequent in the nadroparin than in the citrate group ($p < 0.001$). In this study, hospital mortality and mortality at 3 months were unexpectedly reduced in the citrate group in both per-protocol and intention-to-treat analyses. This is a strong finding, as mortality is rarely modified by a single technique in intensive care unit (ICU) patients, and this is the only technique that proved superior among those adopted for CRRT. As survival is rarely modified by interventions in these studies, other surrogate outcomes are commonly used as proxy of safety and performance, including circuit survival time, bleeding and major adverse events, platelet count, and discontinuation of CRRT for bleeding.

Several other strategies have been developed to minimize filter clotting during CRRT. One is predilution, without circuit anticoagulation that prolongs circuit survival and is a safe approach in critically ill patients at high risk of bleeding [5]. This technique has the advantage of avoiding any form of anticoagulation, reducing bleeding complications. However, so far it is not clear which category of patients can truly benefit from predilution without anticoagulation, as most critically ill patients are non-bleeding or not at high risk of bleeding. This technique can indeed reduce circuit lifespan, consequently increasing costs and reducing CVVH efficacy. Moreover, predilution reduces CRRT efficacy, as uremic toxins and other substances are diluted in blood before CRRT filter, and it is not the best available option when higher CRRT doses are needed.

As mentioned, systemic anticoagulation with unfractionated heparin (UH) is the most common strategy employed during CVVH. Several randomized controlled trials have compared UH and regional citrate anticoagulation [2, 4, 6, 7]. A meta-analysis of randomized trials, published in 2012, found a decreased risk of bleeding in patients treated with citrate, but no difference in survival [8]. Other studies found that a reduced bleeding risk with citrate anticoagulation as compared with systemic heparin is achieved without reducing or even increasing clotting-free circuit survival time [9, 10]. However, despite a lower complication rate, no difference in mortality was identified when comparing UH and citrate anticoagulation [9].

Several studies compared the efficacy and safety of UH and LMWH. A similar rate of bleeding, circuit survival, and platelet consumption was found. No significant difference in mortality was identified for these treatments [11, 12].

In conclusion, citrate has proven to be superior to LMWH on mortality, while no definitive conclusion can be drawn from studies comparing citrate and UH. However, considering that UH was not proven superior to LMWH in terms of mortality in several studies, and that citrate showed a reduced complication rate when compared with UH, citrate may be considered at least as safe, and probably safer, than UH in terms of mortality. Further randomized studies with larger sample size are needed for a definitive answer.

7.3 Pathophysiological Principles

Blood flow through the extracorporeal circuit directly triggers coagulation, due to the contact with artificial surfaces and with air in the bubble trap, to turbulent and low flow, and to hemoconcentration. Citrate is a well-known anticoagulant. It has been used for decades as an anticoagulant to preserve stored blood products. Indeed, citrate chelates calcium ions, a necessary cofactor in the coagulation cascade, thus reducing calcium levels. The reduced calcium concentration hampers thrombin generation, the fundamental final step of intrinsic and extrinsic pathways in the coagulation cascade.

The citrate-calcium complex is removed from the circuit through hemofiltration and dialysis, while normal calcium levels are restored through a post-filter calcium infusion. This normally grants regional anticoagulation within the extracorporeal circuit, with low risk of bleeding in most patients.

The local extracorporeal effect of citrate anticoagulation is the main principle behind its safety. All other anticoagulants are administered and exert their effects systemically, causing complications in every organ. In patients at high risk of bleeding, anticoagulants are used at a lower dose to reduce complications. However, this strategy may reduce CRRT circuit lifespan. Conversely, during citrate regional anticoagulation blood clotting is impaired only in the CRRT circuit, as citrate is infused and removed (for the largest part) before blood reinfusion to the patient. Metabolic and ionic derangements due to the small amount of citrate that enters systemic circulation are easily monitored and reversible using point of care analyzers.

7.4 Therapeutic Use

The main indication for citrate regional anticoagulation is CRRT in critically ill patients at high risk of bleeding.

The number needed to treat to prevent one bleeding event with citrate regional anticoagulation was calculated to be 6.87 [8, 13]. While citrate CRRT presents higher direct costs than other standard dialytic techniques, citrate anticoagulation was demonstrated to be eventually cheaper than systemic UH, due to increased circuit survival and due to a reduced transfusion and complication rate [14, 15].

The advantages and the indications for the different anticoagulation strategies are summarized in Table 7.1.

Clinicians should consider, during citrate anticoagulation, that despite the removal of most citrate-calcium complex within the dialytic circuit, a small amount of citrate may be delivered to the patient. This can have profound consequences on systemic acid-base balance. Citrate is normally cleared by the liver, almost independently from renal function. Citrate is metabolized in the hepatocytes through Krebs

Table 7.1 Common anticoagulation techniques used for continuous renal replacement therapy

Anticoagulation	Indications	Advantages	Effect on survival
Regional citrate anticoagulation	Patients at high risk of bleeding	Lower risk of bleeding	Citrate reduces mortality against LMWH (nadroparin)
Systemic unfractionated heparin anticoagulation	Critically ill patients	Most used, low costs, easily reversible	None demonstrated
Low molecular weight heparin	Critically ill patients	Low cost, easy to use	Increases mortality when compared to citrate regional anticoagulation in patients at risk of bleeding
Predilution (no anticoagulants)	Patients at high risk of bleeding	No risk of bleeding	None demonstrated

cycle, liberating three molecules of carbon dioxide that are then converted to bicarbonate. Thus, citrate may act as a buffer in the systemic circulation, possibly leading to metabolic alkalosis.

Although trisodium citrate is the primary citrate form in commercial solutions for CRRT, in some cases a small amount of citric acid is added in the preparation. This enhances the anticoagulation effect and reduces the risk of metabolic alkalosis as citric acid is not metabolized to bicarbonate. Moreover, the risk of hypernatremia due to trisodium citrate is reduced by citric acid use.

Citrate may accumulate in patients with hepatic dysfunction, resulting in metabolic acidosis and hypocalcemia. This is the direct consequence of an impairment in citrate metabolism due to liver failure. Acidosis may also occur due to continuous loss of bicarbonate and calcium/citrate complex in the filtrate fluid. The most frequent and dangerous complication is the development of systemic calcium derangements that may be life threatening. Moreover, other electrolytes are chelated by citrate, including phosphorus and magnesium. Therefore, calcium and electrolyte levels should be monitored closely in clinical practice to reduce citrate toxicity.

Liver failure is a relative contraindication for citrate regional anticoagulation, as it implies a higher risk of citrate toxicity. However, citrate anticoagulation can be used even in patients with liver failure if needed, with closer metabolic monitoring [16–18]. Citrate metabolism may be impaired in other conditions with systemic hypoperfusion causing reduced liver blood flow and reduced citrate clearance, such as cardiogenic shock or septic shock. To increase the safety of this technique, standardized local protocols should be employed [13]. Moreover, new commercial solutions and more accurate algorithms for citrate management are being developed to simplify citrate anticoagulation, to reduce the risk of metabolic derangements, and to widen its use in clinical practice [19].

In conclusion, considering the lower risk of complications and some evidence of survival advantage for citrate anticoagulation, the addition of new technological improvements and the evidence of similar total costs, citrate use for CRRT in critically ill patients should probably be increased in the next future. New clinical trials are warranted to definitively assess the effect of citrate anticoagulation in terms of survival benefits, complication rate, and cost-effectiveness.

Clinical Summary

Technique	Indications	Cautions	Side effects	Dose	Notes
Citrate in CRRT	Need for renal replacement therapy in critically ill patients at risk of bleeding	Liver failure, shock	Citrate intoxication, especially in liver failure, leading to hypocalcemia and/or other electrolyte disturbances Acid bases disturbances, including metabolic alkalosis and acidosis	Citrate solution is infused in the arterial line, at 102 mmol/L The rate of calcium chloride reinfused through venous line (starting at 0.5 mL/min) is modified according to calcium levels monitoring	Calcium and other electrolytes levels should be closely monitored to avoid the risk of hypocalcemia Acid-base status should be monitored to avoid acidosis and alkalosis

References

1. Rimes-Stigare C, Frumento P, Bottai M et al (2015) Evolution of chronic renal impairment and long-term mortality after de novo acute kidney injury in the critically ill; a Swedish multicentre cohort study. Crit Care Lond Engl 19:221
2. Hetzel GR, Schmitz M, Wissing H et al (2011) Regional citrate versus systemic heparin for anticoagulation in critically ill patients on continuous venovenous haemofiltration: a prospective randomized multicentre trial. Nephrol Dial Transplant 26(1):232–239
3. Landoni G, Bove T, Székely A et al (2013) Reducing mortality in acute kidney injury patients: systematic review and international web-based survey. J Cardiothorac Vasc Anesth 27(6):1384–1398
4. Oudemans-van Straaten HM, Bosman RJ, Koopmans M et al (2009) Citrate anticoagulation for continuous venovenous hemofiltration. Crit Care Med 37(2):545–552
5. Tan HK, Baldwin I, Bellomo R (2000) Continuous veno-venous hemofiltration without anticoagulation in high-risk patients. Intensive Care Med 26(11):1652–1657

6. Kutsogiannis DJ, Gibney RTN, Stollery D, Gao J (2005) Regional citrate versus systemic heparin anticoagulation for continuous renal replacement in critically ill patients. Kidney Int 67(6):2361–2367
7. Monchi M, Berghmans D, Ledoux D et al (2004) Citrate vs. heparin for anticoagulation in continuous venovenous hemofiltration: a prospective randomized study. Intensive Care Med 30(2):260–265
8. Wu MY, Hsu YH, Bai CH et al (2012) Regional citrate versus heparin anticoagulation for continuous renal replacement therapy: a meta-analysis of randomized controlled trials. Am J Kidney Dis Off J Natl Kidney Found 59(6):810–818
9. Betjes MGH, van Oosterom D, van Agteren M, van de Wetering J (2007) Regional citrate versus heparin anticoagulation during venovenous hemofiltration in patients at low risk for bleeding: similar hemofilter survival but significantly less bleeding. J Nephrol 20(5):602–608
10. Gattas DJ, Rajbhandari D, Bradford C et al (2015) A randomized controlled trial of regional citrate versus regional heparin anticoagulation for continuous renal replacement therapy in critically Ill adults. Crit Care Med 43(8):1622–1629
11. Joannidis M, Kountchev J, Rauchenzauner M et al (2007) Enoxaparin vs. unfractionated heparin for anticoagulation during continuous veno-venous hemofiltration: a randomized controlled crossover study. Intensive Care Med 33(9):1571–1579
12. Reeves JH, Cumming AR, Gallagher L et al (1999) A controlled trial of low-molecular-weight heparin (dalteparin) versus unfractionated heparin as anticoagulant during continuous venovenous hemodialysis with filtration. Crit Care Med 27(10):2224–2228
13. Tolwani A, Wille KM (2012) Regional citrate anticoagulation for continuous renal replacement therapy: the better alternative? Am J Kidney Dis 59(6):745–747
14. Oudemans-van Straaten HM (2014) Citrate for continuous renal replacement therapy: safer, better and cheaper. Crit Care Lond Engl 18(6):661
15. Schilder L, Nurmohamed SA, Bosch FH et al (2014) Citrate anticoagulation versus systemic heparinisation in continuous venovenous hemofiltration in critically ill patients with acute kidney injury: a multi-center randomized clinical trial. Crit Care Lond Engl 18(4):472
16. De Vico P, Messino V, Tartaglione A et al (2015) Safety and efficacy of citrate anti-coagulation continuous renal replacement therapies in post-cardiac surgery patients with liver dysfunction. Ther Apher Dial 19(3):272–278
17. Slowinski T, Morgera S, Joannidis M et al (2015) Safety and efficacy of regional citrate anticoagulation in continuous venovenous hemodialysis in the presence of liver failure: the Liver Citrate Anticoagulation Threshold (L-CAT) observational study. Crit Care 19:349
18. Lahmer T, Messer M, Rasch S et al (2015) Sustained low-efficiency dialysis with regional citrate anticoagulation in medical intensive care unit patients with liver failure: a prospective study. Crit Care 30(5):1096–1100
19. Broman M, Klarin B, Sandin K et al (2015) Simplified citrate anticoagulation for CRRT without calcium replacement. ASAIO J 61(4):437–442

Peri-angiography Hemofiltration to Reduce Mortality

8

Giancarlo Marenzi, Nicola Cosentino, and Antonio L. Bartorelli

8.1 General Principles

One of the most important and well-known complications of contrast agent administration is kidney toxicity and contrast-induced nephropathy (CIN). The incidence of CIN is growing, largely due to the increasing number of cardiac catheterizations and percutaneous coronary interventions (PCI) in elderly patients with associated co-morbidities, such as chronic kidney disease (CKD), diabetes and cardiac failure [1]. The available literature has consistently shown that patients who develop CIN have a greater risk of death, both during hospitalization and for up to one year or more after the contrast-enhanced procedure. Therefore, as CIN is potentially preventable, prophylactic measures are mandatory.

Despite a large number of studies, most of the evaluated prophylactic pharmacologic agents have not proven to be effective, particularly when hard end points are considered. Renal replacement therapies (RRTs) are emerging as useful therapeutic strategies in patients with coexisting cardiovascular and renal pathologies, and they have recently been a matter of deep investigation also in the setting of CIN prevention. This interest lies on the notion that contrast media, due to their relatively small size, lack of protein binding and small volume of distribution, are well suited for removal with RRT [2].

G. Marenzi, MD, FESC (✉) • N. Cosentino, MD
Centro Cardiologico Monzino, via Parea 4, Milan 20138, Italy
e-mail: giancarlo.marenzi@ccfm.it; nicola.cosentino@ccfm.it

A.L. Bartorelli, MD, FESC, FACC
Centro Cardiologico Monzino, via Parea 4, Milan 20138, Italy

Cardiovascular Section, Department of Clinical Sciences and Community Health, University of Milan, Milan, Italy
e-mail: antonio.bartorelli@ccfm.it

© Springer International Publishing Switzerland 2016

G. Landoni et al. (eds.), *Reducing Mortality in Acute Kidney Injury*,
DOI 10.1007/978-3-319-33429-5_8

In this chapter, the potential applications of RRT and, in particular, of hemofiltration, in CIN prevention in patients undergoing PCI, will be discussed on the basis of investigational experiences, with an emphasis on their impact on prognosis.

8.2 Main Evidence

The features and findings of the main studies investigating the prophylactic use of RRT to prevent CIN and to reduce mortality are summarized in Table 8.1.

Hemodialysis was first proposed for CIN prevention after contrast agent administration in patients with CKD, but no clear benefit over hydration, or even potential harm, was demonstrated [3–6]. Indeed, a higher likelihood to have a decline in renal function with additional hemodialysis treatment was reported [4]. Even when hemodialysis was started immediately before contrast agent administration, it did not demonstrate any appreciable protection against CIN [7]. These initial negative results were confirmed in a systematic review [8] and in a more recent meta-analysis [9] that showed no benefit of hemodialysis in CIN incidence as compared to routine preventive care, with, again, a trend toward a greater risk for hemodialysis need [8]. Nevertheless, subgroup analyses found that hemodialysis had a beneficial effect over the standard treatment in reducing the risk of CIN in patients with stage 4 or stage 5 CKD [9]. Consistently, Lee et al. [10] demonstrated the benefit in renal outcome of a 4-h hemodialysis session after coronary angiography in patients with stage 5 CKD. However, hard end points, such as in-hospital and long-term mortality, do not seem to be favourably affected by the use of prophylactic hemodialysis [9, 11].

Continuous hemofiltration, by effectively removing fluid and solute with fluid volume control, is associated with a better hemodynamic stability. Thus, it represents an advantage over high-intensity hemodialysis sessions, especially in the treatment of patients with associated renal and cardiac failure. In 2003, a single-centre randomized controlled trial found that the use of pre-emptive hemofiltration, initiated 4–8 h before contrast exposure and continued for 18–24 h after the procedure, resulted in a significant reduction of CIN incidence (5 % vs. 50 %) and in an improved in-hospital (2 % vs. 18 %) and 1-year (10 % vs. 30 %) mortality in patients with severe CKD undergoing elective PCI [1]. A subsequent randomized study, comparing the use of saline hydration with pre- and post-procedural hemofiltration or the use of post-procedural hemofiltration only in severe CKD patients scheduled for elective procedures, concluded that pre- and post-hemofiltration was superior to the other two strategies, in terms of CIN incidence, in-hospital clinical complications, and mortality [12]. In line with these findings, it has been recently demonstrated, in 46 CKD patients undergoing PCI, that hemofiltration (if serum creatinine <3 mg/dL) or hemodiafiltration (if serum creatinine >3 mg/dL) performed before and after contrast medium administration was more effective in preventing a further worsening of renal function as compared to post-procedural treatment only. Moreover, at 18 months, a significantly lower overall mortality was observed in patients treated with RRT pre-post vs. RRT post (16 % vs. 57 %) [13]. However, in

Table 8.1 Summary of studies on the prophylactic use of renal replacement therapy to prevent contrast-induced nephropathy and to reduce mortality

Source	Type of study	Number of patients	Type of procedure	RRT modality	Protocol			CIN prevention	Mortality reduction
					Before CE	After CE	Qr/Qd		
Lehnert (1998) [5]	Prospective randomized	30	Angiography	HD	–	3 h	Qd 500 mL/min	No	–
Sterner (2000) [3]	Prospective randomized	32	Angiography	HD	–	4 h	NA	No	–
Vogt (2001) [4]	Prospective randomized	113	Renal PTA Peripheral PTA CT scan CA	HD	–	3 h	Qd 500 mL/min	No	–
Frank (2003) [7]	Prospective randomized	17	CA	HD	–	4 h	Qd 500 mL/h	No	–
Marenzi (2003) [1]	Prospective randomized	114	Elective CA and PCI	HF	4–6 h	18–24 h	Qr 1,000 mL/h	Yes	Yes
Marenzi (2006) [12]	Prospective randomized	92	Coronary angiography + PCI	HF HF	6 h	18–24 h 18–24 h	Qr 1,000 mL/h	Yes Yes	Yes Yes
Lee (2007) [10]	Prospective randomized	82	CA Elective PCI Urgent PCI	HD	–	4 h	Qd 500 mL/min	Yes	–
Reinecke (2007) [11]	Prospective randomized	424	Elective CA	HD	–	2 h	Qd 500 mL/min	No	No
Ghani (2011) [15]	Prospective Observational	98	CA PCI	HF		18–24 h	Qr 2,000 mL/h	Yes	–

(continued)

Table 8.1 (continued)

Source	Type of study	Number of patients	Type of procedure	RRT modality	Protocol			CIN prevention	Mortality reduction
					Before CE	After CE	Qr/Qd		
Spini (2013) [13]	Prospective Observational	46	Elective PCI Urgent PCI Emergent PCI	HD/HDF	6 h	18–24 h 18–24 h	Qr 1,000 mL/h Qd 1,000 mL/h	Yes Pre-post vs. post	Yes Pre-post vs. post
Choi (2014) [16]	Prospective randomized	68	CA Elective and urgent PCI	HF	During CA		Qr 2,000 mL/h	Yes	–
Guastoni (2014) [17]	Prospective Observational	53	CA Elective PCI Urgent PCI	HF		6 h	Qr 25 mL/min	Yes	–
Marenzi (2015) [18]	Prospective Observational	60	Urgent and emergent PCI	HDF		3 h	Qr 2,000 mL/h Qd 30 L/h	Yes	Yes

CA coronary angiography, *CE* contrast exposure, *CIN* contrast-induced nephropathy, *HD* hemodialysis, *HF* hemofiltration, *HDF* hemodiafiltration, *NA* not available, *PCI* percutaneous coronary intervention, *PTA* percutaneous transluminal angioplasty, *Qd* dialysate pump rate, *Qr* replacement rate, *RRT* renal replacement therapy

a recent meta-analysis including 11 trials (9 randomized and 2 nonrandomized), although hemofiltration and haemodiafiltration were found to significantly reduce the risk of acute temporary RRT, their use did not affect CIN occurrence and did not improve mortality [9].

Although the notion that a pre-procedural RRT session is required in order to obtain a full clinical benefit, its use before coronary angiography and PCI is unsuitable for many patients with acute coronary syndrome (ACS), who often need an emergency or urgent intervention. In addition, ACS patients represent a population at high risk of CIN, given the large amount of contrast that may be required, the frequently associated hemodynamic instability and the preclusion from adequate CIN prophylaxis measures before contrast exposure [14]. In 2011, Saudi et al. [15] demonstrated that a 24-h hemofiltration session, performed as soon as possible after contrast injection in 98 CKD patients undergoing coronary angiography, resulted in a very low CIN incidence (1 %). However, since a clinical follow-up was not available, the potential prognostic implications of hemofiltration could not be determined. In a subsequent study, hemofiltration performed only during coronary intervention in CKD patients, with stable and unstable (about 40 %) coronary artery disease, provided a similar protection against CIN occurrence and a better 30-day renal outcome using significantly less medical resources as compared to peri-procedural hemofiltration, suggesting that simultaneous hemofiltration can be immediately performed in patients undergoing emergency coronary intervention [16]. In agreement with these preliminary data, Guastoni et al. [17] demonstrated that hemofiltration performed for 6 h after a diagnostic or interventional coronary procedure in patients with severe CKD, also including those with ACS, was able to remove more than half of the administered contrast medium. Again, this was associated with a low incidence of CIN. A recent study evaluated such a strategy in high-risk ACS patients with associated severe renal and cardiac dysfunction, undergoing urgent or primary PCI and found that a 3-h treatment with haemodiafiltration, initiated immediately after PCI, significantly impacted on in-hospital (3 % vs. 23 %) and 1-year mortality (10 % vs. 53 %) [18]. Of note, the incidence of stage 2–3 acute kidney injury (10 % vs. 40 %) and the need for rescue RRT (7 % vs. 27 %) during hospitalization were significantly lower among haemodiafiltration-treated patients, suggesting that the possible clinical benefit associated with haemodiafiltration could have been driven by the marked reduction in the occurrence rate of severe acute kidney injury.

8.3 Pathophysiological Principles

A possible explanation for the lack of a beneficial effect associated with the use of hemodialysis is that, by inducing hypovolemia, it may worsen renal ischemic injury, delay recovery of renal function and result in a need for prolonged treatment. On the other hand, continuous hemofiltration is associated with hemodynamic stability and, by preserving the volume of circulating blood, it safeguards against renal hypoperfusion. This effect is particularly useful when coronary procedures are performed in patients with critical conditions. In addition to hemodynamic stability, hemofiltration provides controlled high-volume hydration and removal of contrast agent from the circulation, with a resultant reduction in the kidneys' exposure to the agent. It can also be speculated that, in addition to high-volume controlled hydration, the removal by convective filtration and by adsorption to the filter membrane of mediators of contrast-induced toxicity, such as endothelin, angiotensin, prostaglandins and adenosine, as well as of uremic toxins, may play an additional protective role during the hemofiltration session preceding contrast exposure. Finally, a renal protective effect may also derive from the alkalinizing bicarbonate-based solution, used in the replacement fluid during hemofiltration.

8.4 Therapeutic Use

Taken together, these data indicate that hemofiltration represents an important advance for CIN prevention, because it allows us to extend the range of patients with advanced CKD who were previously excluded from cardiac catheterization, despite their high coronary atherosclerotic burden, and who may currently undergo invasive cardiovascular procedures safely. However, although a growing amount of data seems to support its use, there is still insufficient evidence to confirm a routine employment of hemofiltration for both CIN prevention and outcome improvement in clinical practice in high-risk patients [19]. Accordingly, the most recent guidelines on myocardial revascularization of the European Society of Cardiology and the European Association for Cardio-Thoracic Surgery have recommended (Class IIa recommendation, level of evidence B) the use of prophylactic hemofiltration for prevention of CIN only in patients with severe CKD undergoing complex PCI [20].

In conclusion, the role of these therapies in the highest risk patients, namely, those with associated cardio-renal dysfunction, where adequate intravenous hydration may be difficult and fraught with complications, seems to be promising. As only patients with very low residual renal function seem to benefit from these therapies, they should be the focus of studies that wish to test the potential clinical

Clinical Summary

Strategy	Indications	Side effects	Dose
Peri-angiography hemofiltration	Complex PCI in severe CKD patients	*Related to vascular access* (haemorrhage, infection, insertion complication) *Related to heparinization* (haemorrhage, thrombocytopenia)	Prophylactic 6 h before PCI continued for 24 h after the procedure Fluid replacement rate 1,000 mL/h without negative loss and saline hydration

advantage of RRT. Therefore, future studies are warranted to better define the specific role of these approaches, with particular emphasis on hard clinical end points, optimally customized prophylactic protocols and their most cost-effective application.

References

1. Marenzi G, Marana I, Lauri G et al (2003) The prevention of radiocontrast-agent-induced nephropathy by hemofiltration. N Engl J Med 349:1331–1338
2. Cruz DN, Perazella MA, Ronco C (2008) The role of extracorporeal blood purification therapies in the prevention of radiocontrast-induced nephropathy. Int J Artif Organs 31:515–524
3. Sterner G, Frennby B, Kurkus J et al (2000) Does post-angiographic hemodialysis reduce the risk of contrast medium nephropathy? Scand J Urol Nephrol 34:323–326
4. Vogt B, Ferrari P, Schonholzer C et al (2001) Prophylactic hemodialysis after radiocontrast media in patients with renal insufficiency is potentially harmful. Am J Med 111:692–698
5. Lehnert T, Keller E, Gondolf K et al (1998) Effect of hemodialysis after contrast medium administration in patients with renal insufficiency. Nephrol Dial Transplant 13:358–362
6. Kawashima S, Takano H, Iino Y et al (2006) Prophylactic hemodialysis does not prevent contrast-induced nephropathy after cardiac catheterization in patients with chronic renal insufficiency. Circ J 70:553–558
7. Frank H, Werner D, Lorusso V et al (2003) Simultaneous hemodialysis during coronary angiography fails to prevent radiocontrast-induced nephropathy in chronic renal failure. Clin Nephrol 60:176–182
8. Cruz DN, Perazella MA, Bellomo R et al (2006) Extracorporeal blood purification therapies for prevention of radiocontrast-induced nephropathy: a systematic review. Am J Kidney Dis 48:361–371
9. Cruz DN, Goh CY, Marenzi G et al (2012) Renal replacement therapies for prevention of radiocontrast-induced nephropathy: a systematic review. Am J Med 125:66–78
10. Lee PT, Chou KJ, Liu CP et al (2007) Renal protection for coronary angiography in advanced renal failure patients by prophylactic hemodialysis. A randomized controlled trial. J Am Coll Cardiol 50:1015–1020
11. Reinecke H, Fobker M, Wellmann J et al (2007) (2007) A randomized controlled trial comparing hydration therapy to additional hemodialysis or N-acetylcysteine for the prevention of contrast medium-induced nephropathy: the Dialysis-versus-Diuresis (DVD) Trial. Clin Res Cardiol 96:130–139
12. Marenzi G, Lauri G, Campodonico J et al (2006) Comparison of two hemofiltration protocols for prevention of contrast-induced nephropathy in high-risk patients. Am J Med 119:155–162
13. Spini V, Cecchi E, Chiostri M et al (2013) Effects of two different treatments with continuous renal replacement therapy in patients with chronic renal dysfunction submitted to coronary invasive procedures. J Invasive Cardiol 25:80–84
14. Marenzi G, Lauri G, Assanelli E et al (2004) Contrast-induced nephropathy in patients undergoing primary angioplasty for acute myocardial infarction. J Am Coll Cardiol 44:1780–1785
15. Ghani AA, Hussain N, Al Helal B (2011) Can continuous venovenous hemofiltration prevent contrast-agent induced nephropathy in patients with advanced chronic kidney disease after coronary angiography? Saudi J Kidney Dis Transpl 22:54–60
16. Choi MJ, Yoon JW, Han S et al (2014) The prevention of contrast-induced nephropathy by simultaneous hemofiltration during coronary angiographic procedures: a comparison with periprocedural hemofiltration. Int J Cardiol 176:941–945
17. Guastoni C, Bellotti N, Poletti F et al (2014) Continuous venovenous hemofiltration after coronary procedures for the prevention of contrast-induced acute kidney injury in patients with severe chronic renal failure. Am J Cardiol 113:588–592

18. Marenzi G, Mazzotta G, Londrino F et al (2015) Post-procedural hemodiafiltration in acute coronary syndrome patients with associated renal and cardiac dysfunction undergoing urgent and emergency coronary angiography. Catheter Cardiovasc Interv 85:345–351
19. Landoni G, Bove T, Székely A et al (2013) Reducing mortality in acute kidney injury patients: systematic review and international web-based survey. J Cardiothorac Vasc Anesth 27:1384–139
20. Windecker S, Kolh P, Alfonso F et al (2014) 2014 ESC/EACTS guidelines on myocardial revascularization: the task force on myocardial revascularization of the European Society of Cardiology (ESC) and the European Association for Cardio-Thoracic Surgery (EACTS) developed with the special contribution of the European Association of Percutaneous Cardiovascular Interventions (EAPCI). Eur Heart J 35:2541–2619

9 Continuous Venovenous Hemofiltration to Reduce Mortality in Severely Burned Patients

Kevin K. Chung

9.1 General Principles

Among severely burned patients who require hospitalization, the prevalence of acute kidney injury (AKI) has been reported to be close to 25 %, with an associated mortality of 35 % [1]. Among those who require renal replacement therapy (RRT), the reported mortality is up to 80 %, and it is likely higher than in the non-burn critically ill population (60 %) [1, 2]. It is presumable that this high associated mortality is closely tied to burn size and age and thus relatively non-modifiable. However, recent studies suggest that it is possible to alter survival in this patient population with an early, aggressive approach to RRT. More importantly, the traditional approach of waiting for classically taught triggers for the initiation of RRT (such as refractory acidosis, severe electrolyte abnormalities, intoxication with dialyzable substances, intractable fluid overload, and uremic complications such as pericarditis and encephalopathy) may result in an unacceptably high mortality [3].

The specific mode of RRT also deserves careful consideration for the treatment of AKI in burned patients. Convective solute clearance through hemofiltration-based RRT has theoretical advantages in the setting of an augmented immune/inflammatory state, due to the nonspecific removal of middle molecular weight mediators (10–50 kDa) [4]. In contrast, solute diffusion with reliance on concentration gradients through hemodialysis-based RRT only effectively targets small molecules. The contrast between continuous and intermittent modes of RRT and their corresponding clinical implications is also of interest in the burn population. It is commonly accepted that continuous modes are better tolerated from a hemodynamic standpoint than intermittent therapies [5, 6]. Additionally, continuous therapies may be associated with better long-term outcomes as defined by less need for long-term dialysis among survivors [7, 8].

K.K. Chung, MD, FCCM
US Army Institute of Surgical Research, Fort Sam Houston, TX, USA
e-mail: kevin.k.chung.mil@mail.mil

© Springer International Publishing Switzerland 2016

G. Landoni et al. (eds.), *Reducing Mortality in Acute Kidney Injury*,
DOI 10.1007/978-3-319-33429-5_9

Therefore, a reasonable argument can be made for continuous venovenous hemofiltration (CVVH) as the mode of choice for severe burns with AKI. A recent systematic review revealed only one study suggesting that this intervention improves mortality [9]. This study and its implications will be reviewed in this chapter.

9.2 Main Evidence

Early reported experience in burns by Leblanc et al. [10] suggested that continuous renal replacement therapy (CRRT) was hemodynamically well tolerated while providing good metabolic and volume control. Their reported mortality rate was however 82 %, similarly to other reports, which also showed high mortality rates among burn patients treated with CRRT [11–14].

In a study comparing early aggressive CRRT in burned military casualties, a decreased in-hospital mortality from 88 % to 56 % was demonstrated when comparing a treated group to a historical control of patients who were managed using the conservative approach of waiting for traditional dialysis indications [14]. Of note, none of the patients in the conservative arm survived long enough to meet the criteria for dialysis, and thus, none were offered any form of RRT. When the sample size was nearly doubled with the addition of civilian burn patients treated in the same facility, the improvement in survival was sustained [15]. Again, only a small fraction of patients in the conservative arm (2/28) received any form of RRT, suggesting that applying traditional dialysis initiation criteria in burns only leads to an unacceptably high death rate. Interestingly, a significant improvement in hemodynamic parameters was observed among those who were placed on CVVH while in shock ($n=21$), with most of them being completely weaned off vasopressor support within 48 h. Additionally, patients with acute respiratory distress syndrome (ARDS) had a significant improvement in oxygenation within 24 h from CVVH initiation ($n=16$).

This study certainly has some limitations: the sample size is small, the study is retrospective and it is from a single center. Therefore, caution should be applied when interpreting these findings into actual practice. Accordingly, the first web-enabled international consensus conference on mortality reduction in patients with or at risk for AKI recently recommended against the routine application of CVVH in severely burned patients with the intent of increasing survival [9]. Nonetheless, it is important to individualize interventions based on the best available evidence when dealing with a niche population such as burns, where robust populations do not readily exist for the purposes of large randomized multicenter studies. In fact, if on the one hand the impact of this specific therapy on survival in burn patients with AKI is probably unclear, on the other hand, an unacceptably high mortality is almost certain if no therapy is applied in this setting.

9.3 Pathophysiological Principles

Treatment of burn patients with CVVH resulted in an observed improvement in hemodynamics and lung function [15]. This suggests a potential extrarenal benefit. Hemodynamic improvement has been observed in other studies where a relatively high dose of replacement volumes has been used [16]. In the discussed study on CVVH in burned patients, the mean hemofiltration dose prescribed was 57 ± 19 mL kg^{-1} h^{-1} [15]. This dosage places this technique in the "high-volume hemofiltration" category, capable of removing circulating mediators and cytokines from the blood compartment, as demonstrated in numerous preclinical studies [16]. The profoundly dysregulated inflammatory host response observed in the critically ill burn population may thus be ideally suited for this type of approach [17]. Regardless, it is not possible to attribute any potential benefit to an aggressively applied (high-volume) mode of therapy (hemofiltration) in the right population (burns) as early application (timing) may also be a factor.

High-volume hemofiltration (70 mL kg^{-1} h^{-1}) applied in a critically ill population was not found to be superior to a lower dose of hemofiltration (35 mL kg^{-1} h^{-1}) in a randomized controlled trial [18]. Caution should be applied in the extrapolation of these findings to the burn population.

Obviously, more carefully designed studies are needed. However, while the optimal mode and dose of therapy in burns continue to be up for debate, it is clear that waiting for "traditional" dialysis indications only leads to an unacceptably high mortality rate in this unique population. Early and aggressive application of some form of RRT regardless of mode and dose may be better than waiting for arbitrary and absolute triggers.

9.4 Therapeutic Use

Application of CVVH, especially higher doses, comes with some unique practical considerations. Some of these have been mentioned in the Clinical Summary. First, as with any mode of RRT, regular monitoring of electrolytes is a must. In particular, given that the convective approach can remove larger molecules in the middle molecular weight range, extra attention should be paid to avoidance of hypophosphatemia. Second, the mode and dose of therapy, along with native renal clearance, need to be taken into account when determining appropriate doses of therapeutic drugs such as antimicrobials [19]. Finally, when applying a higher hemofiltration dose by increasing the replacement fluid rate, careful consideration of the filtration fraction is needed, and blood flow must be increased accordingly to avoid early clogging of the filter [20]. In general, a filtration fraction less than 25 % is desired to maintain adequate filter patency. This can be achieved by increasing the blood flow rate of the circuit along with the replacement fluid rate.

Clinical Summary

Technique	Indications	Cautions	Side effects	Dose	Notes
CVVH	AKI in burns	Dose adjustment of antimicrobials needed	Electrolyte depletion Loss of micronutrients	20–35 mL kg^{-1} h^{-1}	Early initiation may be beneficial
High-volume hemofiltration	AKI in burns with septic shock	Dose adjustment of antimicrobials needed	Electrolyte depletion Loss of micronutrients	>35 mL kg^{-1} h^{-1}	Evidence in the general critically ill population suggests no benefit Appears to be safe

References

1. Brusselaers N, Monstrey S, Colpaert K et al (2010) Outcome of acute kidney injury in severe burns: a systematic review and meta-analysis. Intensive Care Med 36:915–925
2. Uchino S, Kellum JA, Bellomo R et al (2005) Acute renal failure in critically ill patients: a multinational, multicenter study. JAMA 294:813–818
3. Irwin RS, Rippe JM (2008) Irwin and Rippe's intensive care medicine. Lippincott Williams & Wilkins, Philadelphia, pp 988–999
4. Linden K, Stewart IJ, Kreyer SFX et al (2014) Extracorporeal blood purification in burns: a review. Burns 40:1071–1078
5. Kidney Disease: Improving Global Outcomes (KDIGO) Acute Kidney Injury Work Group (2012) KDIGO clinical practice guideline for acute kidney injury. Kidney Inter Suppl 2:1–138
6. Palevsky PM, Zhang JH, O'Connor TZ, for the VA/NIH Acute Renal Failure Trial Network et al (2008) Intensity of renal support in critically ill patients with acute kidney injury. N Engl J Med 359:7–20
7. Gallagher M, Cass A, Bellomo R et al (2014) Long-term survival and dialysis dependency following acute kidney injury in intensive care: extended follow-up of a randomized controlled trial. PLoS Med 11:e1001601
8. Palevsky PM, O'Connor TZ, Chertow GM et al (2009) Intensity of renal replacement therapy in acute kidney injury: perspective from with the Acute Renal Failure Trial Network Study. Crit Care 13:310
9. Landoni G, Bove T, Szekely A et al (2013) Reducing mortality in acute kidney injury patients: systematic review and international web-based survey. JCVA 27:1384–1398
10. Leblanc M, Thibeault Y, Querin S (1997) Continuous haemofiltration and haemodiafiltration for acute renal failure in severely burned patients. Burns 23:160–165
11. Holm C, Horbrand F, von Donnersmarck GH, Muhlbauer W (1999) Acute renal failure in severely burned patients. Burns 25:171–178
12. Triolo G, Mariano F, Stella M et al (2002) Dialytic therapy in severely burnt patients with acute renal failure. G Ital Nefrol 19:155–159

13. Hladik M, Tymonava J, Zaoral T et al (2001) Treatment by continuous renal replacement therapy in patients with burn injuries. Acta Chir Plast 43:21–25
14. Chung KK, Juncos LA, Wolf SE et al (2008) Continuous renal replacement therapy improves survival in severely burned military casualties with acute kidney injury. J Trauma 64:S179–S187
15. Chung KK, Lundy JB, Matson JR et al (2009) Continuous venovenous hemofiltration in severely burned patients with acute kidney injury: a cohort study. Crit Care 13:R62
16. Honore PM, Joannes-Boyau O, Boer W, Collin W (2009) High-volume hemofiltration in sepsis and SIRS: current concepts and future prospects. Blood Purif 28:1–11
17. Jeschke MG, Chinkes DL, Finnerty CC et al (2008) Pathophysiologic response to severe burn injury. Ann Surg 248:387–401
18. Joannes-Boyau O, Honore PM, Bagshaw SM et al (2013) High-volume versus standard-volume haemofiltration for septic shock patients with acute kidney injury (IVOIRE study): a multicentre randomized controlled trial. Intensive Care Med 39:1535–1546
19. Choi G, Gomersall CD, Tian Q et al (2009) Principles of antibacterial dosing in continuous renal replacement therapy. Crit Care Med 37:2268–2282
20. Joannidis M, Straaten O (2007) Clinical review: patency of the circuit in continuous renal replacement therapy. Crit Care 11:218

10 Perioperative Hemodynamic Optimization to Reduce Acute Kidney Injury and Mortality in Surgical Patients

Nicola Brienza, Mariateresa Giglio, and Argentina Rosanna Saracco

10.1 General Principles

Each year, 234 millions major surgical procedures are performed worldwide. Despite the overall low risk of death and complications, over 80 % of postoperative deaths occur in a specific high-risk subgroup of patients in whom an imbalance between global oxygen delivery (DO_2) and oxygen consumption (VO_2) develops [1]. This derangement derives from a complex interplay between surgery-induced inflammatory response and patient status, with an increased oxygen demand [2, 3] that sometimes fails to be matched by an adequate increase in DO_2, thus leading to hypoperfusion and tissue hypoxia. The consequences of tissue hypoxia include the activation of both endothelium, leading to capillary leak, and pro-inflammatory cytokines, leukocytes, and complement cascade, enhancing the inflammatory status. If this process is untreated, fatal postoperative complications may develop [4].

Postoperative acute kidney injury (AKI) affects 1–37 % of patients after surgery [5, 6]. Its occurrence is associated with higher rates of gastrointestinal bleeding, respiratory infections, and sepsis [7, 8]. Very recent evidences show that the risk-adjusted average cost of care for patients undergoing surgery is $42,600 for patients with any stage of AKI compared with $26,700 for patients without AKI and the risk-adjusted 90-day mortality is 6.5 % for patients with any stage of AKI compared with 4.4 % for patients without AKI [9].

N. Brienza, MD, PhD (✉) • M. Giglio, MD
Anesthesia and Intensive Care Unit, Department of Emergency and Organ Transplantation, University of Bari, Piazza G. Cesare, 11, Bari 70100, Italy
e-mail: nicola.brienza@uniba.it; mariateresagiglio@gmail.com

A.R. Saracco, MD
Intensive Care And Anesthesia Division, Azienda Ospedaliera ASL Taranto, Polo Occidentale, Italy
e-mail: a_saracco@libero.it

© Springer International Publishing Switzerland 2016

G. Landoni et al. (eds.), *Reducing Mortality in Acute Kidney Injury*,
DOI 10.1007/978-3-319-33429-5_10

Several risk factors have been associated with postoperative AKI. Most of these are non-modifiable, either procedure related (urgent surgery, need for surgical re-exploration, cardiopulmonary bypass duration) or patient related (age >70 years, diabetes mellitus, atrial fibrillation, left ventricular dysfunction, preoperative intra-aortic balloon pump counterpulsation, chronic renal failure) [5]. Cardiovascular surgery is, by far, the surgical procedure with the higher risk of postoperative AKI, with up to 30 % of patients experiencing AKI [5], although a recent retrospective study suggests that the incidence of postoperative AKI in noncardiac surgery may be quite close (22.4 %) [10]. This study shows that postoperative AKI is independently associated with increased in-hospital mortality (patients who developed AKI were 3.7 times more likely to die); moreover, the more severe AKI, the higher in-hospital mortality. In addition to severity, the duration of AKI may be a predictor of in-hospital mortality. A recent observational study stratifies postsurgical patients with AKI according to the maximum KDIGO class (see Chap. 2) and the duration of AKI, showing a significant increase (2.5 %) in hospital mortality for each extra day of AKI duration for those episodes lasting <2 weeks [11].

Therefore, improving the renal outcome of high-risk surgical patients is of considerable clinical importance, especially as it may favorably influence survival and improve resource allocation. Nevertheless, there are still a lot of uncertain aspects due to the absence of a homogeneous definition of AKI, of renal risk stratification, and of studies with adequate power and appropriate sample composition.

10.2 Pathophysiology

Historically, the mechanisms of AKI have been classified as prerenal, intrinsic, and postrenal. Ischemic forms, prerenal azotemia, and acute tubular necrosis are the most common causes of AKI in hospitalized patients. However, AKI represents a continuum of injury, and the distinction between prerenal azotemia and acute tubular necrosis is likely not reflective of tubular biology. Postoperative AKI may involve prerenal factors and progress toward acute tubular necrosis through acute ischemic or toxic injuries [12]. The underlying mechanism is multifactorial: hemodynamic, inflammatory, and nephrotoxic factors may be all involved, and overlap each other, in causing kidney injury. Moreover, the type of surgery, coexisting diseases, and preoperative renal function are critical risk factors, alone or in synergetic association [12–14]. Additionally, a surgery-related inflammatory response with activation of the cytokine network, reactive oxygen species (ROS) formation, and leukocyte infiltration may contribute to kidney injury.

The multifactorial pathogenesis of AKI probably explains why evidence-based preventive strategies are still lacking. In 2005, a systematic review did not find any reliable evidence from the available literature to suggest that drugs such as dopamine, diuretics, calcium channel blockers, or angiotensin-converting enzyme inhibitors can exert a renal protective action [15]. Aimed to improve outcome in critically ill patients with AKI, a set of guidelines was released by the Kidney Disease: Improving Global Outcomes (KDIGO) group in 2012 and recently updated [16].

This group of experts stated that hemodynamic optimization with isotonic crystalloids and vasopressors is the cornerstone for prevention of AKI, together with avoiding iodinated contrast and other nephrotoxic drugs.

Hemodynamic optimization, also known as goal-directed therapy (GDT), refers to the monitoring and manipulation of physiological hemodynamic parameters by means of various therapeutic interventions, including the administration of fluids, but also of red blood cells and inotropic drugs, aimed to face the increase in oxygen demand. Since 1988 (when Shoemaker et al. [17] performed the first interventional trial on perioperative GDT), several investigations have been performed with conflicting results. Subsequent meta-analyses [18, 19], considering separately surgical and septic/critically ill patients, confirmed that mortality was improved only in the perioperative setting. The beneficial effect of GDT only in surgical patients may rely on the basis that, while in the early stage of systemic inflammatory response syndrome it is possible to prevent the deleterious effects of oxygen debt, when the inflammatory process has advanced oxygen debt is no longer reversible and increasing oxygen transport is no longer effective. The reduction in mortality observed with GDT seems to be related to the reduction in perioperative morbidity, including renal injury.

10.3 Main Evidence

A recent meta-analysis of 20 studies (including 4,220 patients, overall) specifically addressed the potential nephroprotective role of perioperative targeted hemodynamic optimization with fluids and/or inotropes, showing that GDT decreased the risk of postoperative renal impairment (Table 10.1) [20]. Interestingly, both intraoperative and postoperative optimizations were as much effective as preoperative optimization. Accordingly, from a "renal standpoint," hemodynamic optimization performed during or soon after surgery seems to be a feasible alternative when preoperative optimization is difficult to pursue. Moreover, targeting the optimization to physiological values of cardiac output has proven to be as much nephroprotective as adopting "supranormal goals" (e.g., DO_2 index >600 mL min^{-1} m^{-2}, or cardiac index >4.5 L min^{-1} m^{-2}). Nevertheless, due to the potential risk of complications such as fluid overload, myocardial ischemia, as well as further deterioration of renal function [21], both an aggressive administration of fluids and an excessive use of catecholamines, in the attempt to increase cardiac output to supranormal values, should be avoided. Other subgroup analyses demonstrated the beneficial effect of GDT in high-risk patients, when fluids and inotropes were used together to reach hemodynamic targets and when a pulmonary artery catheter (PAC) was used as compared with less-invasive monitoring tools. The latter analyses, however, were limited by low statistical power, and no definitive conclusions can be drawn about these issues.

These findings were confirmed by a subsequent systematic review, demonstrating the ability of the association of fluids and inotropes to reach hemodynamic goals and reduce postoperative AKI [22]. Moreover, this paper suggested that GDT may reduce postoperative AKI not only by providing extra fluid when indicated but also

Table 10.1 Subgroup analyses of pooled OR of renal injury in perioperative hemodynamic goal-directed studies

	Treatment (*n*/*N*)	Control (*n*/*N*)	OR (95 % CI)	*p* value		I^2 (%)	Statistical power (%)
Quality of RCTs (Jadad score ≥3)	102/1741	150/1699	0.66 (0.50–0.87)	0.003	0.75	0	99.7
Preoperative optimization	94/1347	117/1289	0.70 (0.53–0.94)	0.02	0.41	0	75.6
Intraoperative or postoperative optimization	21/770	58/814	0.47 (0.27–0.81)	0.006	0.80	0	100
High-risk patients	102/1393	158/99.8	0.64 (0.49–0.84)	0.001	0.53	0	99.8
Non high-risk patients	13/724	17/686 1	0.69 (0.31–1.54	0.37	0.61	0	19.1
Pulmonary artery catheter monitoring	103/1640	151/1629	0.62 (0.43–0.90	0.01	0.35	10.3	98
Other monitoring devices	12/477	24/474	0.52 (0.25–1.07)	0.07	0.87	0	73
Fluids only	6/334	12/333	0.55 (0.20–1.47)	0.23	0.74	0	31
Fluids + inotropes	109/1783	163/1770	0.65 (0.50–0.85)	0.002	0.50	0	100
Fluids + dobutamine	12/511	42/518	0.36 (0.18–0.75)	0.006	0.57	0	100
Supranormal targets	30/354	55/353	0.49 (0.29–0.83)	0.008	0.54	0	98.2
Normal targets	85/1763	120/1750	0.70 (0.52–0.94)	0.02	0.71	0	94.5

Adapted from Brienza et al. [20]
OR odds ratio, *CI* confidence interval, *RCT* randomized controlled trial

by allowing earlier and guided use of fluids and by preventing the administration of unnecessary fluids when hemodynamic target is met.

In a recent international, web-enabled consensus conference, dealing with the interventions that may influence survival in critically ill patients with or at risk for AKI, GDT was graded as 1C (i.e., strong recommendation supported by low quality of evidence; see Chap. 3) [23]. Interestingly, GDT received a 100 % agreement by the consensus meeting and a 97 % agreement by the web voters worldwide, resulting in the most suggested recommendation in order to reduce mortality in critically ill patients with or at risk for AKI.

At the moment, GDT is the only approach that can be endorsed in order to reduce the incidence of postoperative AKI. GDT may decrease the risk of postoperative renal injury by assuring adequate renal blood flow and reducing renal vasoconstriction. Moreover, thanks to the reduced risk of renal hypoxia, this strategy may attenuate a vicious cycle of destructive processes, including inflammation, differentiation, fibrosis, peritubular capillary narrowing, impaired renal autoregulation, oxidative stress, apoptosis, and necrosis.

10.4 Clinical Considerations

Interventions to optimize hemodynamics are diverse in nature, targets, timing, design, and technology (see Table 10.1). This heterogeneity leads to uncertainty about the precise nature of treatments and/or technologies that should be applied to achieve hemodynamic optimization. For example, different studies on GDT varied their approach regarding the type of fluid used to reach hemodynamic targets, since some trials used crystalloids, while others used only colloids. Recent evidence suggests that the type of fluid is also likely important in determining renal function [24]. Several concerns about renal toxicity of starch-based solutions, in fact, have been raised in the ICU population, and their safety in surgical patients is still under debate [25–27] (See Chap. 20). Similarly, high-chloride fluids are suggested to exert an adverse effect on renal function [24, 28]. Moreover, even if evidence shows that the use of inotropes after fluid loading may confer significant benefits, it is not possible to state whether the effects of fluid and inotropes are synergistic or whether the beneficial effect of one intervention counteracts the adverse effect of the other. So far there is no a "best" monitoring tool or hemodynamic target, and the choice of perioperative hemodynamic monitoring for GDT depends on both surgery-related and patient-related risks. Empirically, patients with cardiac morbidity undergoing major surgical interventions which imply large fluid shifts and hemodynamic stress would draw maximum benefit from more invasive monitoring (e.g., pulmonary artery catheter), but limited evidence exists. Specific trials investigating these issues are still lacking.

Conclusion

AKI is a serious complication in surgical and critical care patients and carries an increased risk of mortality and additional hospital costs. One advantage with postoperative AKI is that the moment of the actual insult to the kidney is known,

Clinical Summary

Strategy	Indications	Cautions	Side effects	Dose	Notes
Perioperative hemodynamic optimization	Surgical patients at high risk for perioperative morbidity/mortality	Monitoring tools and variables to be targeted should be properly chosen according to the patient and the type of surgery	Possible fluid overload, myocardial ischemia, and further deterioration of renal function	Fluid and inotropes in appropriate doses to achieve normal values of certain hemodynamic variables (e.g., CI 2.5–4 $L/min/m^2$ and DO_2I 500–600 $mL/min/m^2$)	Colloids and high-chloride fluids should be used with caution The highest is the patient-related or surgery-related risk, the more invasive should be the monitoring adopted

and this should facilitate the use of adequate preventive strategies. Nevertheless, evidence-based recommendations to prevent postsurgical AKI are still scarce. Recent evidence demonstrates that hemodynamic optimization to reduce mortality in critically ill patients with or at risk for AKI is supported by high-level evidence. Several points of debate are, however, still open, including the type of fluid to be used to reach the hemodynamic targets, the inotropic support, the choice of the monitoring tool as well as of the hemodynamic variables to be targeted, and which subgroup of the high-risk surgical population could benefit most from a GDT approach. Forthcoming trials are needed to clarify whether using less-invasive monitoring tools and targets may play an effective role in protecting renal function after surgery. Moreover, the role of inotropic support to preserve renal function during surgery needs to be clarified. Finally, prospective RCTs are needed to clarify which perioperative goal-directed fluid strategy may protect and which may even harm renal function.

References

1. Jhanji S, Thomas B, Ely A et al (2008) Mortality and utilisation of critical care resources amongst high-risk surgical patients in a large NHS trust. Anaesthesia 63:695–700
2. Pearse R, Dawson D, Fawcett J, Rhodes A, Grounds RM, Bennett ED (2005) Changes in central venous saturation after major surgery, and association with outcome. Crit Care 9:R694–R699
3. Shoemaker WC, Appel PL, Kram HB (1993) Haemodynamic and oxygen transport responses in survivors and nonsurvivors of high-risk surgery. Crit Care Med 21:977–990
4. Kusano C, Baba M, Takao S et al (1997) Oxygen delivery as a factor in the development of fatal postoperative complications after oesophagectomy. Br J Surg 84:252–257
5. Parolari A, Pesce LL, Pacini D et al (2012) Risk factors for perioperative acute kidney injury after adult cardiac surgery: role of perioperative management. Ann Thorac Surg 93(2):584–591
6. Bihorac A, Brennan M, Basianti T et al (2013) National surgical quality improvement program underestimates the risk associated with mild and moderate postoperative acute kidney injury. Crit Care Med 41:2570–2583
7. Aronson S, Blumenthal R (1998) Perioperative renal dysfunction and cardiovascular anesthesia: concerns and controversies. J Cardiothorac Vasc Anesth 12:567–586
8. Thakar CV, Yared JP, Worley S et al (2003) Renal dysfunction and serious infections after open-heart surgery. Kidney Int 64:239–246
9. Hobson C, Ozrazgat-Baslanti T, Kuxhausen A et al (2015) Cost and mortality associated with postoperative acute kidney injury. Ann Surg 261:1207–1214
10. Teixeira C, Rosa R, Rodrigues N et al (2014) Acute kidney injury after major abdominal surgery: a retrospective cohort analysis. Crit Care Res Pract 2014:132175
11. Wu HC, Wang J, Chen YW, Chen HH (2015) The association between the duration of postoperative acute kidney injury and in-hospital mortality in critically ill patients after non-cardiac surgery: an observational cohort study. Ren Fail 37(6):985–993
12. Carmichael P, Carmichael AR (2003) Acute renal failure in the surgical setting. ANZ J Surg 73:144–153
13. Glodowski SD, Wagener G (2014) New insights into the mechanisms of acute kidney injury in the intensive care unit. J Clin Anesth 27(2):175–180

14. Gomez H, Ince C, De Backer D et al (2014) A unified theory of sepsis-induced acute kidney injury: inflammation, microcirculatory dysfunction, bioenergetics, and the tubular cell adaptation to injury. Shock 41(1):3–11
15. Joannidis M, Druml W, Forni LG et al (2010) Prevention of acute kidney injury and protection of renal function in the intensive care unit: expert opinion of the working group for nephrology, ESICM. Intensive Care Med 36:392–411
16. Hoste E, De Corte W (2013) Implementing the kidney disease: improving global outcomes/acute kidney injury guidelines in ICU patients. Curr Opin Crit Care 19:544–553
17. Shoemaker WC, Appel PL, Kram HB, Waxman K, Lee TS (1988) Prospective trial of supranormal values of survivors as therapeutic goals in high-risk surgical patients. Chest 94(6):1176–1186
18. Hamilton MA, Cecconi M, Rhodes A (2011) A systematic review and meta-analysis on the use of preemptive hemodynamic intervention to improve postoperative outcomes in moderate and high-risk surgical patients. Anesth Analg 112(6):1392–1402
19. Gurgel ST, do Nascimento P (2011) Maintaining tissue perfusion in high-risk surgical patients: a systematic review of randomized clinical trials. Anesth Analg 112(6):1384–1391
20. Brienza N, Giglio MT, Marucci M, Fiore T (2009) Does perioperative hemodynamic optimization protect renal function in surgical patients? A meta-analytic study. Crit Care Med 37(6):2079–2090
21. Heringlake M, Wernerus M, Grunefeld J et al (2007) The metabolic and renal effects of adrenaline and milrinone in patients with myocardial dysfunction after coronary artery bypass grafting. Crit Care 11:R51
22. Prowle JR, Chua HR, Bagshaw SM, Bellomo R (2012) Clinical review: volume of fluid resuscitation and the incidence of acute kidney injury – a systematic review. Crit Care 16(4):230
23. Landoni G, Bove T, Székely A et al (2013) Reducing mortality in acute kidney injury patients: systematic review and international web-based survey. J Cardiothorac Vasc Anesth 27(6):1384–1398
24. Prowle J, Bellomo R (2013) Fluid administration and the kidney. Curr Opin Crit Care 19:308–314
25. Heßler M, Arnemann PH, Ertmer C (2015) To use or not to use hydroxyethyl starch in intraoperative care: are we ready to answer the 'Gretchen question'? Curr Opin Anaesth 28(3):370–377
26. Yates DR, Davies SJ, Milner HE, Wilson RJ (2014) Crystalloid or colloid for goal-directed fluid therapy in colorectal surgery. Br J Anaesth 112(2):281–289
27. Feldheiser A, Pavlova V, Bonomo T, Jones A, Fotopoulou C, Sehouli J, Wernecke KD, Spies C (2013) Balanced crystalloid compared with balanced colloid solution using a goal-directed haemodynamic algorithm. Br J Anaesth 110(2):231–240
28. Krajewski ML, Raghunathan K, Paluszkiewicz SM, Schermer CR, Shaw AD (2015) Meta-analysis of high- versus low-chloride content in perioperative and critical care fluid resuscitation. Br J Surg 102(1):24–36

11 Furosemide by Continuous Infusion to Reduce Mortality in Patients with Acute Kidney Injury

Michael Ibsen and Anders Perner

11.1 General Principles

In critically ill patients admitted to an intensive care unit (ICU), there is a high incidence of both oliguric and non-oliguric acute kidney injury (AKI). Many patients also receive fluid resuscitation, and this, especially in combination with oliguric AKI, carries a high risk of clinically significant fluid overload. Fluid overload (defined as an overall accruement of fluid by more than 10 % of baseline body weight) is associated with higher mortality, longer duration of mechanical ventilation and greater ICU length of stay [1–3]. The exact pathogenesis leading to adverse outcome following fluid overload is not known in detail, but tissue and organ oedema, causing impairment of transport and exchange of oxygen and nutrients, might contribute. Hence, there is great interest in understanding what strategies may be effective in avoiding, or at least mitigating, this potentially harmful condition.

Treatment with diuretics to facilitate the achievement of an even or negative fluid balance, and potentially to prevent the need for renal replacement therapy (RRT), in the setting of AKI has been the subject of great interest. However, the latest international guidelines recommend not using diuretics to prevent or treat AKI (grade 1B, i.e. strong recommendation based on moderate-quality evidence), except in the

M. Ibsen
Department of Intensive Care, Copenhagen University Hospital, Rigshospitalet, Copenhagen DK-2100, Denmark
e-mail: Michael.Ibsen@regionh.dk

A. Perner, MD, PhD (✉)
Department of Intensive Care, Copenhagen University Hospital, Rigshospitalet, Copenhagen DK-2100, Denmark

Department of Intensive Care 4131, Copenhagen University Hospital, Rigshospitalet, Blegdamsvej 9, Copenhagen DK-2100, Denmark
e-mail: anders.perner@rh.regionh.dk

© Springer International Publishing Switzerland 2016

G. Landoni et al. (eds.), *Reducing Mortality in Acute Kidney Injury*,
DOI 10.1007/978-3-319-33429-5_11

management of fluid overload (grade 2C, i.e. weak recommendation with low- or very low-quality evidence) [4].

Furosemide is a loop diuretic and can be administered intravenously both as bolus injections and as a continuous infusion. We examined the evidence from several randomised clinical trials (RCTs) and one meta-analysis of RCTs comparing the effects of administration of furosemide as a continuous infusion vs. bolus administration in the setting of AKI with and without fluid overload. Furosemide use in the setting of primary heart failure is beyond the scope of this chapter.

11.2 Main Evidence

11.2.1 Evidence from Randomised Clinical Trials

The first group who investigated the use of furosemide as continuous infusion was Copeland and colleagues [5]. They randomly assigned 18 cardiac surgery patients (9 in each group) to receive 0.3 mg/kg furosemide as a bolus injection or 0.05 mg kg^{-1} h^{-1} as an infusion. There were no differences between groups after 12 h, but continuous infusion provided less variable and more sustained diuresis from hour to hour.

Schuller et al. [6] enrolled 33 cardiac and medical ICU patients with pulmonary oedema or fluid overload. The patients were randomised to either bolus or continuous administration of furosemide titrated to achieve an average hourly net negative fluid balance of at least 1 mL/kg, but no differences were observed between the groups.

In 2002, Martin et al. [7] investigated both continuous furosemide and albumin infusion, as compared with placebo, in hypoproteinaemic patients with acute lung injury. Thirty-seven mechanically ventilated patients from two university hospitals were included. No mortality difference was seen, but the albumin-furosemide group had improved diuresis and weight loss (on average, 5.3 kg more over 5 days, $p=0.04$), as well as better oxygenation and haemodynamic variables, as compared to the placebo group.

Mojtahedzadeh et al. [8] randomised 22 medical ICU patients with pulmonary oedema or fluid overload. Consistently with the findings of Schuller et al. [6], furosemide administration as either a bolus or continuous infusion was equally effective in achieving a negative fluid balance.

In 2007, Ostermann et al. [9] compared the two regimens in 59 patients with fluid overload in two general ICUs. They found no difference in hospital mortality, frequency of mechanical ventilation, changes in serum creatinine or estimated glomerular filtration rates. However, the total dose of furosemide was significantly lower in the continuous infusion group (9 mg/h vs. 24 mg/h, $p<0.001$), and urine output per mg furosemide was higher in the continuous infusion group (31.6 vs. 18 mL/mg, $p=0.01$).

The most recent and also the largest study was that by Kunt et al. [10]. These investigators randomised 100 patients with normal renal function undergoing elective coronary bypass surgery to either of the two dosing regimens. In the bolus group, urine output was significantly lower and the use of RRT was higher ($p=0.03$). Also, mortality was higher in the bolus group (7 patients vs. 1 died, $p=0.03$). This is, so far, the only investigation reporting a survival benefit with continuous infusion of furosemide as compared to bolus administration. However, it has been criticised for important methodological flaws [11].

In summary, three of the studies comparing furosemide by continuous infusion with bolus administration reported on mortality. Two studies found no difference [7, 9], whereas one low-quality study found a reduced mortality with continuous infusion [10]. There is weak evidence that continuous furosemide infusion is more effective in achieving larger diuresis and better control of fluid balance, without large fluctuations in blood volume, as compared to bolus administration [9–11]. However, some studies found similar effects between the two regimes. We found no studies specifically designed to investigate the role of continuous furosemide infusion in prevention of sepsis-associated AKI or to assess the influence of continuous furosemide infusion on outcomes in septic patients with AKI.

11.2.2 Systematic Reviews and Meta-analyses

We found only one systematic review with meta-analysis specifically focusing on furosemide as a continuous infusion versus bolus injection [12]. This review included comparative trials of furosemide bolus vs. continuous infusion by random allocation in surgical or ICU patients. Four trials including a total of 129 patients were included in the analysis. Furosemide as continuous infusion was not associated with a significant reduction in the risk of hospital mortality as compared to bolus administration (odds ratio [OR] 0.60, 95 % confidence interval [CI] 0.20–1.84, $p=0.37$). Thus, existing data are insufficient to recommend a better way to administer furosemide which could impact mortality, as well as other patient-relevant outcome measures or resource use.

11.3 Pharmacologic Properties

Furosemide is a loop diuretic and acts primarily by inhibiting the Na-K-2Cl cotransport in the thick ascending limb of the loop of Henle, thus reducing NaCl reabsorption. In theory, loop diuretics as a group have several effects that could protect against AKI (see also Chap. 21). They may decrease oxygen consumption, both in the loop of Henle and in renal tubules, by inhibiting sodium transport, thereby potentially preventing or attenuating ischaemic injury [13, 14]. Moreover, as shown in an experimental study in dogs, furosemide could reduce renovascular resistance and increase renal blood flow, thus washing out necrotic debris that block renal tubules, an effect that might hasten recovery from AKI or at least reduce its severity [15].

However, these theoretically beneficial pharmacological effects have never been shown to translate into clinical benefits. There is no evidence that the use of diuretics reduces the rate or severity of AKI [16]. Similarly, the potential advantages of continuous infusion, such as a more effective fluid balance control without large fluctuations in circulating volume, that may even worsen kidney injury (see also Chap. 19) have not been shown so far to provide a survival benefit in critically ill patients with AKI.

11.4 Therapeutic Use

Typical indications for administration of furosemide in the ICU setting are oliguria in adequately fluid-resuscitated patients, induction of diuresis in patients with severe fluid overload and achievement of a negative fluid balance in patients with severe lung injury.

Usual doses are 5–20 (or 40) mg bolus injections intravenously in patients with presumed or known normal renal function, while higher doses (80–250 mg) can be used in patients with known impairment of renal function, especially in those with chronic kidney disease.

Infusion doses are typically in the range of 5–40 mg/h or approximately 0.05–0.5 mg kg^{-1} h^{-1}.

Following intravenous administration, the effect sets in after 5 min and the plasma half-life varies from 30 min to 2 h.

Contraindications include known allergy, hypovolaemia or dehydration and anuria. Reported toxic effects are tinnitus or even hearing loss, while common side effects are electrolyte (hypokalaemia, hyponatraemia, hypomagnesaemia) and acid-base disturbances (metabolic alkalosis), dehydration and increases in serum creatinine.

Conclusion

In theory, furosemide has several pharmacological effects that might be beneficial in patients at risk of developing AKI or in patients with established AKI without anuria.

Furosemide can be administered intravenously either as bolus injections or as a continuous infusion. There is weak evidence that continuous furosemide infusion is more effective in achieving larger diuresis and better control of fluid balance as compared to bolus administration. However, there are no data from high-quality trials indicating that continuous infusion of furosemide prevents AKI or reduces its severity, nor that improves survival in critically ill patients.

Clinical Summary

Drug/ strategy	Indications	Contraindications	Side effects	Dose	Notes
Furosemide by continuous infusion	Fluid overload (oliguria despite fluid resuscitation)	Known allergy Anuria Hypovolaemia Dehydration	Hearing loss Tinnitus Electrolyte disturbances Dehydration Increase in serum creatinine	Typically 5–40 mg/h	There is no high-quality evidence supporting a survival benefit with continuous infusion of furosemide in AKI patients

References

1. Vaara ST, Korhonen AM, Kaukonen KM et al (2012) Fluid overload is associated with an increased risk for 90-day mortality in critically ill patients with renal replacement therapy: data from the prospective FINNAKI-study. Crit Care 16:R197
2. Bouchard J, Soroko SB, Chertow GM et al (2009) Fluid accumulation, survival and recovery of kidney function in critically ill patients with acute kidney injury. Kidney Int 76(4):422–427
3. de Oliveira FS, Freitas FG, Ferreira EM et al (2015) Positive fluid balance as a prognostic factor for mortality and acute kidney injury in severe sepsis and septic shock. J Crit Care 30(1):97–101
4. Kidney Disease: Improving Global Outcomes (KDIGO) Acute Kidney Injury Work Group (2012) KDIGO clinical practice guideline for acute kidney injury. Kidney Int Suppl 2(1):1–138
5. Copeland JG, Campbel DW, Plachetka JR et al (1983) Diuresis with continuous infusion of furosemide after cardiac surgery. Am J Surg 146(6):796–799
6. Schuller D, Lynch JP, Fine D (1997) Protocol-guided diuretic management: comparison of furosemide by continuous infusion and intermittent bolus. Crit Care Med 25(12):1969–1975
7. Martin GS, Mangialardi RJ, Wheeler AP et al (2002) Albumin and furosemide therapy in hypoproteinemic patients with acute lung injury. Crit Care Med 30(10):2175–2182
8. Mojtahedzadeh M, Salehifar E, Vazin A et al (2004) Comparison of hemodynamic and biochemical effects of furosemide by continuous infusion and intermittent bolus in critically ill patients. J Infus Nurs 27(4):255–261
9. Ostermann M, Alvarez G, Sharpe MD, Martin CM (2007) Frusemide administration in critically ill patients by continuous compared to bolus therapy. Nephron Clin Pract 107(2):c70–c76
10. Kunt AT, Akgun S, Atalan N et al (2009) Furosemide infusion prevents the requirement of renal replacement therapy after cardiac surgery. Anadolu Kardiyol Derg 9(6):499–504
11. Landoni G, Bove T, Szekely A et al (2013) Reducing mortality in acute kidney injury patients: systematic review and international web-based survey. J Cardiothorac Vasc Anesth 27(6):1384–1398

12. Zangrillo A, Cabrini L, Monti G et al (2011) Continuous infusion versus bolus injection of furosemide in critically ill patients: a systematic review and meta-analysis. Signa Vitae 6:58–63
13. Ponto LL, Schoenwald RD (1990) Furosemide (frusemide) a pharmacokinetic/pharmacodynamic review (part I). Clin Pharmacokinet 18:381–408
14. Ponto LL, Schoenwald RD (1990) Furosemide (frusemide) a pharmacokinetic/pharmacodynamic review (part II). Clin Pharmacokinet 18:460–471
15. Ludens JH, Williamson HE (1970) Effect of furosemide on renal blood flow in the conscious dog. Proc Soc Exp Biol Med 133:513–515
16. Ho KM, Sheridan DJ (2006) Meta-analysis of frusemide to prevent or treat acute renal failure. BMJ 333(7565):420

N-acetylcysteine to Reduce Mortality in Cardiac Surgery

12

Matteo Parotto and Duminda N. Wijeysundera

12.1 General Principles

Acute kidney injury (AKI) is a frequent complication of cardiac surgery, affecting up to 30% of patients [1, 2]. Patients who experience AKI after cardiac surgery have a higher risk for postoperative morbidity, as well as increased short-term and long-term mortality [1, 2]. The important prognostic implications of postoperative AKI have prompted extensive research in the quest to find treatments to reduce mortality in this population. Despite these efforts, there remains a paucity of interventions proven to prevent AKI after cardiac surgery. Most assessed interventions, such as diuretics, low-dose dopamine, and mannitol, have shown minimal, if any benefit, in small randomized controlled trials [3]. A few other interventions (e.g., fenoldopam, off-pump cardiac surgery) showed promise in initial small trials [4, 5] but then failed to confirm these benefits in larger multicenter trials [6, 7].

M. Parotto, MD, PhD
Department of Anesthesia and Pain Management, Toronto General Hospital, Eaton Wing 3-438, 200 Elizabeth Street, Toronto M5G 2C4, ON, Canada

Department of Anesthesia, University of Toronto, Toronto, ON, Canada
e-mail: matteo.parotto@uhn.ca

D.N. Wijeysundera, MD, PhD, FRCPC (✉)
Department of Anesthesia and Pain Management, Toronto General Hospital, Eaton Wing 3-450, 200 Elizabeth Street, Toronto M5G 2C4, ON, Canada

Department of Anesthesia, University of Toronto, Toronto, ON, Canada

Li Ka Shing Knowledge Institute of St. Michael's Hospital, Toronto, ON, Canada

Institute of Health Policy Management and Evaluation, University of Toronto, Toronto, ON, Canada
e-mail: d.wijeysundera@utoronto.ca

© Springer International Publishing Switzerland 2016

G. Landoni et al. (eds.), *Reducing Mortality in Acute Kidney Injury*,
DOI 10.1007/978-3-319-33429-5_12

12.2 Pharmacologic Properties

AKI after cardiac surgery is likely multifactorial in etiology, with several different underlying mechanisms of injury [8]. These mechanisms include ischemic renal injury, reduced nitric oxide activity, and oxygen-free radical injury due to ischemia-reperfusion, cardiopulmonary bypass, nephrotoxins, or reduced plasma glutathione concentration. *N*-acetylcysteine (NAC) has the potential to inhibit several of these mechanisms [9], in that it directly scavenges free radicals, improves blood flow through nitric oxide-mediated pathways, and functions as a precursor for glutathione synthesis.

While there is physiological rationale for NAC being able to prevent postoperative AKI, it is likely that the major impetus for its application in cardiac surgery was due to the initial promising data in the setting of contrast-induced nephropathy. In 2000, Tepel and colleagues [10] published a small placebo-controlled randomized trial on 83 participants in which prophylactic oral administration of NAC significantly reduced AKI rates in patients with chronic renal failure receiving intravenous radiographic contrast agents. Their initial promising results led to numerous subsequent studies that evaluated the effects of different doses and formulations of NAC in the prevention of contrast-induced nephropathy. Despite the early enthusiasm, the benefits of NAC for preventing contrast-induced nephropathy were not consistently replicated in subsequent small trials [11], meta-analyses of such trials [12], or a single large multicenter trial involving 2308 participants [13]. Furthermore, doubts have been raised about the artifactual effect of NAC on biochemical assays for creatinine, which may have explained the positive results seen in some trials [14].

12.3 Main Evidence

Analogous to the evolution of evidence for the efficacy of *N*-acetylcysteine to prevent contrast-induced nephropathy, conflicting results have also emerged from research into its efficacy for preventing perioperative AKI in cardiac surgery patients. In general, research to date has identified no major consistent clinical benefits of NAC in cardiac surgery.

A recent meta-analysis (see Table 12.1) showed that the perioperative use of NAC has no proven benefit for clinically important outcomes in patients undergoing cardiac surgery, such as death or need for renal replacement therapy (RRT) [15]. In meta-regression analyses, treatment effects on AKI were not related to the dose of *N*-acetylcysteine. In addition, no significant differences were found between the NAC and placebo groups with respect to the risks of increase in serum creatinine concentration by 25 % or greater above baseline, acute myocardial infarction, atrial fibrillation, stroke, infection, intra-aortic balloon pump (IABP) support, vasopressor or inotropic support, prolonged mechanical ventilation, length of mechanical ventilation, intensive care unit (ICU) stay, or hospital length of stay [15].

Consistent with the findings of this meta-analysis, a recent web-based international consensus conference issued only a weak recommendation for NAC as a treatment to improve survival in patients undergoing cardiac surgery [16].

Table 12.1 Summary of a recent meta-analysis regarding the use of *N*-acetylcysteine in cardiac surgery [15]

Characteristics of studies included	Number of studies included	Total number of patients included in the meta-analysis	Median dose of *N*-acetylcysteine	Clinical outcomes		
				Incidence of acute renal failure	All-cause mortality	Side effects
Adult patients undergoing cardiac surgery Randomized allocation to *N*-acetylcysteine or placebo groups Reporting at least one relevant clinical or economic outcome	15	1407	9425 mg (range 2400–34,950 mg)	No significant difference between groups	No significant difference between groups	No evidence of significant side effects from *N*-acetylcysteine was reported

The basis for even a weak recommendation was a small single-center randomized controlled trial that found a survival benefit with NAC treatment in 177 cardiac surgery patients with moderate preexisting renal failure [17]. In this study, Wijeysundera and colleagues evaluated a high-dose intravenous *N*-acetylcysteine regimen (100 mg/kg bolus in 30 min after induction of anesthesia, followed by 20 mg kg^{-1} h^{-1} infusion until 4 h after cardiopulmonary bypass) in a randomized placebo-controlled trial where the primary outcome was the percent change in estimated glomerular filtration rate (GFR) during the first 72 postoperative hours [17]. While the authors found no significant effect on the primary outcome, they reported a significant reduction in all-cause mortality among individuals randomized to NAC. These findings should be viewed cautiously since all-cause mortality was a secondary outcome, and there were only seven mortality events in the trial. Furthermore, as indicated previously, these benefits with respect to mortality were not confirmed in subsequent trials and meta-analyses [16].

The absence of consistent benefit has also been observed in recent small randomized trials published after the previously described meta-analysis [15] and consensus conference [16]. For example, in a trial that assessed NAC for preventing AKI in 117 high-risk patients undergoing off-pump coronary artery bypass surgery, Song and colleagues [18] showed no significant benefits of this treatment as compared to placebo. Conversely, Santana-Santos and colleagues [19] reported that high-dose intravenous NAC (150 mg/kg bolus followed by 50 mg/kg infusion for 6 h) reduced the risk of AKI, abolished oxidative stress, and mitigated the negative effect of cardiopulmonary bypass on renal function in 70 patients with chronic kidney disease undergoing

Clinical Summary

Drug/technique	Indications	Cautions	Side effects	Dose	Notes
N-acetylcysteine (NAC)	Patients undergoing cardiac surgery with or without preexisting chronic renal dysfunction (not on preoperative dialysis)	There are some data suggesting that NAC interferes with the usual biochemical assay for creatinine. This finding might explain why measures of renal function sometimes appear better with the use of NAC	Side effects are rare They include anaphylactoid reactions. Increased blood loss and blood product transfusion requirements have been described; however, these side effects were not confirmed by recent meta-analysis	Multiple regimens described, with no proven differences between different protocols Oral 600 mg twice a day from preoperative day 1 to postoperative day 1–5 Intravenous bolus preoperatively/pre-cardiopulmonary bypass (1200 mg intravenous bolus or 50–150 mg/kg) followed by intravenous repeated bolus/infusion for up to 36 h postoperatively Median total dose among trials was 9425 mg (range 2400–34,950 mg)	The findings of several trials and meta-analyses only justify a weak recommendation for considering NAC as a treatment to improve survival in patients undergoing cardiac surgery

coronary artery bypass graft surgery. In contrast to some of the previous studies, Santana-Santos and colleagues offered evidence that NAC abolishes the increase in circulating reactive oxygen species observed in the control group, thus confirming a plausible mechanistic explanation for the observed nephroprotective effect.

12.4 Therapeutic Use

N-acetylcysteine can be administered orally or intravenously. The bioavailability after oral administration is approximately 6–10 %. Renal clearance constitutes 30 % of total body clearance, and the elimination half-life is 2.3 h. Several dosing regimens of NAC for patients undergoing cardiac surgery have been described in the literature. Some protocols included oral administration before and/or after surgery, with doses of 600 mg twice a day for different durations of time (3–7 days, starting preoperatively). Intravenous regimens typically involved a bolus (50–150 mg/kg) before the beginning of surgery, followed by subsequent boluses (600 or 1200 mg every 12 h until 24 or 36 h postoperatively) or infusion of varying doses (from approximately 2–20 mg kg^{-1} h^{-1}) and duration (from until the end of surgery to 48 h postoperatively). The abovementioned recent meta-analysis reported that the median perioperative total dose used in previous studies of NAC in cardiac surgery was 9425 mg (range 2400–34,950 mg) [15].

In general, there are no contraindications to use NAC in cardiac surgery. It is not associated with major adverse effects. High-dose intravenous use, typically exceeding 150 mg/kg, carries the potential risk of anaphylactoid reactions [18]. Chronic systemic NAC administration has been shown to cause pulmonary hypertension in an experimental murine model [16], but no similar effects have been described to date in clinical or acute administration settings. Notably, both Wijeysundera and colleagues [20] and Naughton and colleagues [12] described the potential for NAC to be associated with increased blood loss and blood products transfusion in cardiac surgery patients with preexisting moderate renal failure. Nonetheless, further research did not confirm these findings, with the meta-analysis by Wang and colleagues [15] concluding that NAC had no significant impact on postoperative chest tube drainage, surgical re-exploration, reoperation for bleeding, and red blood cell transfusion requirements.

To date, no major consistent clinical benefits of *N*-acetylcysteine have been identified in the setting of cardiac surgery. There is weak to no evidence for recommending it as a treatment to improve survival in this patient population.

References

1. Pickering JW, James MT, Palmer SC (2015) Acute kidney injury and prognosis after cardiopulmonary bypass: a meta-analysis of cohort studies. Am J Kidney Dis 65(2):283–293
2. Kandler K, Jensen ME, Nilsson JC et al (2014) Acute kidney injury is independently associated with higher mortality after cardiac surgery. J Cardiothorac Vasc Anesth 28(6):1448–1452

3. Park M, Coca SG, Nigwekar SU et al (2010) Prevention and treatment of acute kidney injury in patients undergoing cardiac surgery: a systematic review. Am J Nephrol 31(5):408–418
4. Zangrillo A, Biondi-Zoccai GG, Frati E et al (2012) Fenoldopam and acute renal failure in cardiac surgery: a meta-analysis of randomized placebo-controlled trials. J Cardiothorac Vasc Anesth 26(3):407–413
5. Nigwekar SU, Kandula P, Hix JK, Thakar CV (2009) Off-pump coronary artery bypass surgery and acute kidney injury: a meta-analysis of randomized and observational studies. Am J Kidney Dis 54(3):413–423
6. Garg AX, Devereaux PJ, Yusuf S et al (2014) Kidney function after off-pump or on-pump coronary artery bypass graft surgery: a randomized clinical trial. JAMA 311(21):2191–2198
7. Bove T, Zangrillo A, Guarracino F et al (2014) Effect of fenoldopam on use of renal replacement therapy among patients with acute kidney injury after cardiac surgery: a randomized clinical trial. JAMA 312(21):2244–2253
8. Rosner MH, Okusa MD (2006) Acute kidney injury associated with cardiac surgery. Clin J Am Soc Nephrol 1:19–32
9. Borgström L, Kågedal B, Paulsen O (1986) Pharmacokinetics of N-acetylcysteine in man. Eur J Clin Pharmacol 31(2):217–222
10. Tepel M, van der Giet M, Schwarzfeld C et al (2000) Prevention of radiographic-contrast-agent-induced reductions in renal function by acetylcysteine. N Engl J Med 343(3):180–184
11. Bagshaw SM, McAlister FA, Manns BJ et al (2006) Acetylcysteine in the prevention of contrast-induced nephropathy: a case study of the pitfalls in the evolution of evidence. Arch Intern Med 166:161e6
12. Naughton F, Wijeysundera D, Karkouti K et al (2008) N-acetylcysteine to reduce renal failure after cardiac surgery: a systematic review and meta-analysis. Can J Anaesth 55(12):827–835
13. ACT Investigators (2011) Acetylcysteine for prevention of renal outcomes in patients undergoing coronary and peripheral vascular angiography: main results from the randomized Acetylcysteine for Contrast-induced nephropathy Trial (ACT). Circulation 124(11):1250–1259
14. Hoffmann U, Fischereder M, Kruger B et al (2004) The value of N-acetylcysteine in the prevention of radiocontrast agent-induced nephropathy seems questionable. J Am Soc Nephrol 15:407e10
15. Wang G, Bainbridge D, Martin J, Cheng D (2011) N-acetylcysteine in cardiac surgery: do the benefits outweigh the risks? A meta-analytic reappraisal. J Cardiothorac Vasc Anesth 25(2):268–275
16. Landoni G, Bove T, Székely A et al (2013) Reducing mortality in acute kidney injury patients: systematic review and international web-based survey. J Cardiothorac Vasc Anesth 27(6):1384–1398
17. Wijeysundera DN, Beattie WS, Rao V et al (2007) N-acetylcysteine for preventing acute kidney injury in cardiac surgery patients with pre-existing moderate renal insufficiency. Can J Anesth 54(11):872–881
18. Koppen A, van Riel A, de Vries I, Meulenbelt J (2014) Recommendations for the paracetamol treatment nomogram and side effects of N-acetylcysteine. Neth J Med 72(5):251–257
19. Santana-Santos E, Gowdak LH, Gaiotto FA et al (2014) High dose of N-acetylcysteine prevents acute kidney injury in chronic kidney disease patients undergoing myocardial revascularization. Ann Thorac Surg 97(5):1617–1623
20. Wijeysundera DN, Karkouti K, Rao V et al (2009) N-acetylcysteine is associated with increased blood loss and blood product utilization during cardiac surgery. Crit Care Med 37(6):1929–1934

Fenoldopam and Acute Kidney Injury: Is It Time to Turn the Page?

13

Antonio Pisano, Nicola Galdieri, and Antonio Corcione

13.1 General Principles

First described more than 50 years ago, the use of low-dose dopamine for renal protection (also reported as "renal dose" dopamine) has tenaciously resisted until recently [1, 2]. However, it is now clear that this intervention is, on average, not effective for prevention or early treatment of acute kidney injury (AKI) [1–5] and may even be harmful [5, 6].

Nevertheless, a new enthusiasm has developed during the last decade, although not widely shared [3], for a possible nephroprotective action of fenoldopam, a specific dopamine type-1 receptor (DA_1) agonist which exerts a renal action similar to that of low-dose dopamine, but theoretically more favorable, due to the lack of significant affinity of fenoldopam for DA_2 receptors, and potentially without the adverse effects related to systemic adrenergic stimulation [2, 5, 7, 8]. In particular, two different meta-analyses found a reduction in the need for renal replacement therapy (RRT) and a survival benefit after fenoldopam infusion in patients with or at risk for AKI in different clinical settings [9] and in cardiovascular surgery [10]. Despite it was not possible to recommend its use to prevent or treat AKI according to this evidence [5, 11], fenoldopam remained, until recently, one of the few drugs which were thought to have a potential beneficial effect on renal function, as well as on outcome, in critically ill patients with or at risk for AKI [11–13].

A. Pisano, MD (✉) • N. Galdieri, MD
Cardiac Anesthesia and Intensive Care Unit, A.O.R.N. "Dei Colli" – Monaldi Hospital, via L. Bianchi, Naples 80131, Italy
e-mail: antoniopisanoMD@libero.it; n.galdieri@inwind.it

A. Corcione, MD
Department of Critical Care, A.O.R.N. "Dei Colli", via L. Bianchi, Naples 80131, Italy
e-mail: corcio.ant@libero.it

© Springer International Publishing Switzerland 2016

G. Landoni et al. (eds.), *Reducing Mortality in Acute Kidney Injury*,
DOI 10.1007/978-3-319-33429-5_13

However, the largest multicenter randomized controlled trial (RCT) which addressed the impact of fenoldopam on the need for RRT and on mortality in patients with early cardiac surgery-associated AKI (CSA-AKI) has now been published [8]. As discussed below, its results seriously question the effectiveness (and also the safety) of this strategy.

13.2 Main Evidence

At the time of the first web-enabled international consensus conference on mortality reduction in patients with or at risk for AKI [11], some evidence suggested a potential beneficial role of fenoldopam. The meta-analysis by Landoni and colleagues [9] included 16 RCTs reporting renal outcomes and/or mortality of 1,290 critically ill patients from different clinical settings (cardiac surgery, vascular surgery, liver transplantation, renal transplantation, sepsis, and overall intensive care unit population) randomized to receive fenoldopam or either placebo or best available treatment (mainly low-dose dopamine). Fenoldopam was found to significantly reduce the risk for AKI (odds ratio [OR] 0.43, 95% confidence interval [CI] 0.32–0.59, $p<0.001$), the need for RRT (OR 0.54, 95% CI 0.34–0.84, $p=0.007$), the length of intensive care unit (ICU) stay, and in-hospital mortality (OR 0.64, 95% CI 0.45–0.91, $p=0.01$). A subsequent meta-analysis from the same group focused on cardiovascular surgery patients only but included also case-matched studies in addition to RCTs [10]. Overall, 1,059 patients from 13 studies investigating the role of fenoldopam in both prevention (11 studies) and early treatment (2 studies) of AKI after cardiovascular surgery were analyzed. Once again, a significant reduction in both the need for RRT (OR 0.37, 95% CI 0.23–0.59, $p<0.001$) and in-hospital mortality (OR 0.46, 95% CI 0.29–0.75, $p=0.01$) was shown among patients receiving fenoldopam. A reduction in the ICU length of stay (LOS) was also observed. However, the inclusion in the analysis of studies in which fenoldopam was administered as a prophylactic strategy as well as of studies where fenoldopam was used as a therapeutic intervention, but especially the inclusion of propensity-matched studies rather than only "true" RCTs, represented an important limitation [5].

As highlighted by the authors themselves, most of the trials included in both meta-analyses were of suboptimal quality, and the findings were further limited by the lack of uniform criteria for RRT initiation. Interestingly, although the risk of AKI was still significantly lower in the fenoldopam group after the exclusion, from the first meta-analysis [9], of studies without adequate allocation concealment, statistical significance was lost for the differences in both the need for RRT and mortality.

Indeed, a subsequent updated meta-analysis [14], including only RCTs where fenoldopam was compared with placebo in patients undergoing cardiac surgery, challenged to a certain extent the results of the previous meta-analyses. In fact, Zangrillo and coworkers [14] analyzed 440 patients from 6 RCTs and found a reduced risk of AKI (OR 0.41, 95% CI 0.23–0.74, $p=0.003$) but no differences in the need for RRT, ICU/hospital LOS, or mortality.

Most remarkably, the largest multicenter RCT investigating the role of fenoldopam in the early treatment of CSA-AKI, recently performed by Bove and colleagues

[8] with the aim to shed some light on this limited and in part conflicting evidence, failed to show any benefit from fenoldopam infusion. These authors randomized 667 patients (from 19 cardiac ICUs) who developed RIFLE "R" AKI [15] (see Chap. 2) after cardiac surgery to receive either fenoldopam or placebo. The study was stopped early after a planned interim analysis found no difference in both the need for RRT and 30-day mortality. In particular, 20 % of patients in the fenoldopam group required RRT, as compared with 18 % in the control group ($p=0.47$), while the mortality rate at 30 days was 23 % in the fenoldopam group and 22 % in the placebo group ($p=0.86$). Conversely, a significant increase in the risk of arterial hypotension was found in patients receiving fenoldopam (26 % vs. 15 %, $p=0.01$).

Although it has been objected that an earlier administration of fenoldopam, based on biomarkers allowing an early diagnosis of AKI, could have led to better results [16], a previous high-quality investigation by Bove et al. [17], in which fenoldopam infusion was started after anesthesia induction, did not show any benefit of fenoldopam, as compared with dopamine, on the clinical outcome of CSA-AKI.

13.3 Pharmacologic Properties

The rationale to administer fenoldopam in order to prevent or early treat AKI is similar to the historical reason to use low-dose dopamine: the stimulation of renal DA_1 receptors exerts a natriuretic action and, most importantly, increases global renal blood flow (Fig. 13.1) [2, 4]. DA_1 receptor activates adenylate cyclase, and the resulting increase in cyclic adenosine 3′,5′-monophosphate (cAMP) leads to dilatation of medullary and cortical renal vessels [18], as well as to inhibition of the activity of both apical (e.g., Na^+/H^+ exchange) and basolateral (e.g., Na^+, K^+-ATPase and Na^+/HCO_3^- cotransport) transporters [19].

As previously mentioned, however, it is now clear that dopamine is not effective in improving the outcome of patients with or at risk for AKI [1, 3–5]. It has been thought that the affinity of dopamine also for DA_2 receptors, whose activation inhibits adenylate cyclase, as well as the possibility that even low doses might act on α-adrenergic receptors, causing renal vasoconstriction, may offset the beneficial renal effects of dopamine (see Fig. 13.1). Moreover, dopamine has potential systemic adverse effects, including arrhythmias (e.g., atrial fibrillation/flutter) and myocardial ischemia [5, 6], due to its action on both α- and β-adrenergic receptors.

Fenoldopam is a specific DA_1 agonist with no action on DA_2, α-adrenergic, or β-adrenergic receptors [2, 5, 7, 20]. It is much more potent than dopamine as a renal vasodilator [20]. Moreover, due to its selectivity for DA_1 receptors, fenoldopam increases medullary more than cortical renal blood flow [7], contrarily to dopamine which may cause primarily cortical vasodilation and, accordingly, even worsen medullary ischemia [4]. Finally, fenoldopam is devoid of the adverse effects due to systemic adrenergic stimulation [2, 5, 7]. Despite all these most favorable features, also fenoldopam, as shown above, seems really not to work as a nephroprotective agent.

It has been recently suggested that, especially in patients undergoing cardiac surgery (the surgical setting at higher risk for postoperative AKI [21]), but also in

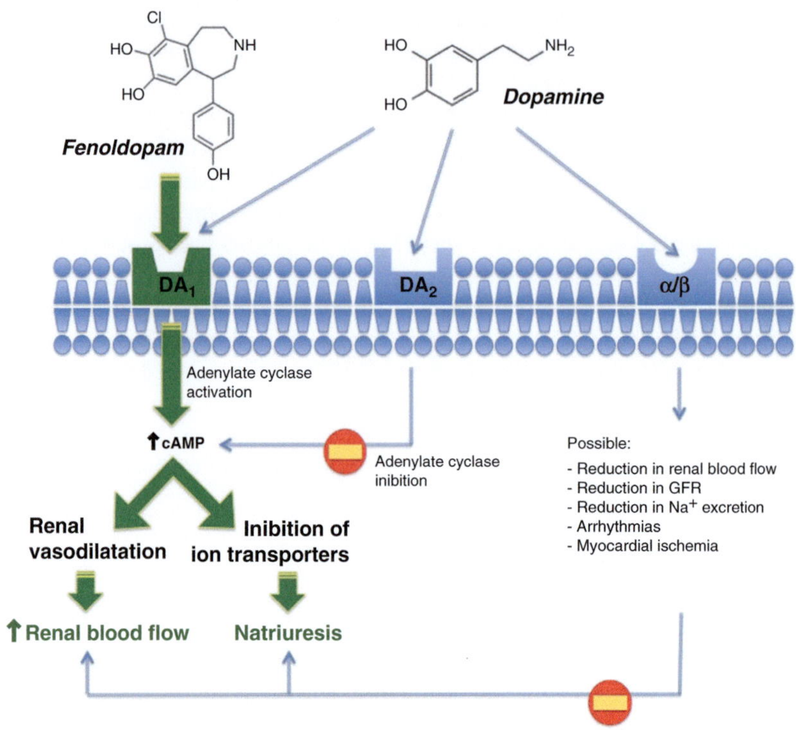

Fig. 13.1 The potentially more favorable "renal" effects of fenoldopam as compared to dopamine. *DA1* dopamine receptor type 1, *DA2* dopamine receptor type 2, *α/β* α- and β-adrenergic receptors, *cAMP* cyclic adenosine 3′,5′-monophosphate, *GFR* glomerular filtration rate

sepsis (the cause of AKI in about one third of ICU patients [22]), the mechanisms of AKI are very rarely purely ischemic, rather involving a strict interplay between inflammation and ischemia/reperfusion injury which leads to the formation of areas of *local* hypoperfusion [2, 3, 16, 23]. Accordingly, simply increasing/restoring global renal blood flow is probably not enough to prevent AKI or its progression toward RRT. Moreover, evidence suggesting an important role of mitochondrial dysfunction in the pathogenesis of AKI is accumulating [24]. Drugs affecting these complex mechanisms may be potentially effective as nephroprotective agents. Actually, some of these drugs are being already studied, with seemingly promising results [2, 24, 25].

13.4 Therapeutic Use

Fenoldopam is a short-acting intravenous antihypertensive drug that reduces systemic vascular resistances in a dose-dependent manner, with an onset time of approximately 5 min and with an action lasting about 30–60 min after discontinuation of infusion [7, 14, 18, 20]. In most studies in which it has been investigated as a nephroprotective

Clinical Summary

Drug	Indications	Cautions	Side effects	Dose	Notes
Fenoldopam	Prevention or early treatment of AKI, especially after cardiac surgery	Adjust dose carefully to avoid hazardous hypotension	Increased risk of hypotension	Around 0.1 μg kg^{-1} min^{-1}	This indication should be probably abandoned

agent, fenoldopam has been administered at a rate of 0.1 μg kg^{-1} min^{-1} [9, 10, 14] for at least 24 h. At this dose, fenoldopam usually increases renal blood flow with no or minimal effects on systemic arterial pressure [7]. However, also the increase in renal blood flow induced by fenoldopam is dose dependent, with the larger increase observed with an infusion rate of 0.3 μg kg^{-1} min^{-1} [19]. In the large multicenter RCT by Bove and colleagues [8], fenoldopam was administered at a mean dose of 0.12 ± 0.06 μg kg^{-1} min^{-1} for a total of 65 ± 30.3 h, with a starting dose of 0.1 μg kg^{-1} min^{-1}, eventually adjusted subsequently, for instance, in case of hypotension.

The main concern when using fenoldopam with the aim to prevent or early treat AKI in surgical or ICU patients is the risk of hypotension, especially when fenoldopam is administered to cardiac surgery patients. The two abovementioned meta-analyses including only cardiac surgery patients [10, 14], as well as the RCT by Bove et al. [8], in fact, reported a significantly increased risk of hypotension. In addiction to be ineffective, therefore, fenoldopam may even be harmful in these patients.

According to the available literature, the level of evidence for the recommendation to not use fenoldopam for AKI treatment or prevention should be upgraded in the next guidelines [4, 5]. At the same time, fenoldopam proved to be a well studied and probably safe drug to be used as an effective vasodilator in the ICU.

References

1. Friedrich JO, Adhikari N, Herridge MS et al (2005) Meta-analysis: low-dose dopamine increases urine output but does not prevent renal dysfunction or death. Ann Intern Med 142(7):510–524
2. Landoni G, Baiardo Redaelli M, Pisano A (2016) Dopamine derivatives and acute kidney injury: the search for the magic bullet continues… and leads to new (magic?) targets. Nephrol Dial Transplant 31(4):512–514
3. Shaw A (2012) Update on acute kidney injury after cardiac surgery. J Thorac Cardiovasc Surg 143(3):676–681
4. Winkelmayer WC, Finkel KW (2014) Prevention of acute kidney injury using vasoactive or antiplatelet treatment: three strikes and out? JAMA 312(21):2221–2222
5. Kellum JA, Lameire N, KDIGO AKI Guideline Work Group (2013) Diagnosis, evaluation, and management of acute kidney injury: a KDIGO summary (part 1). Crit Care 17(1):204

6. Argalious M, Motta P, Khandwala F et al (2005) "Renal dose" dopamine is associated with the risk of new-onset atrial fibrillation after cardiac surgery. Crit Care Med 33:1327–1332
7. Murray PT (2006) Fenoldopam: renal-dose dopamine redux? Crit Care Med 34(3):910–911
8. Bove T, Zangrillo A, Guarracino F et al (2014) Effect of fenoldopam on use of renal replacement therapy among patients with acute kidney injury after cardiac surgery: a randomized clinical trial. JAMA 312(21):2244–2253
9. Landoni G, Biondi-Zoccai GG, Tumlin JA et al (2007) Beneficial impact of fenoldopam in critically ill patients with or at risk for acute renal failure: a meta-analysis of randomized clinical trials. Am J Kidney Dis 49(1):56–68
10. Landoni G, Biondi-Zoccai GG, Marino G et al (2008) Fenoldopam reduces the need for renal replacement therapy and in-hospital death in cardiovascular surgery: a meta-analysis. J Cardiothorac Vasc Anesth 22:27–33
11. Landoni G, Bove T, Székely A et al (2013) Reducing mortality in acute kidney injury patients: systematic review and international web-based survey. J Cardiothorac Vasc Anesth 27(6):1384–1398
12. Landoni G, Augoustides JG, Guarracino F et al (2011) Mortality reduction in cardiac anesthesia and intensive care: results of the first international consensus conference. HSR Proc Intensive Care Cardiovasc Anesth 3(1):9–19
13. Mao H, Katz N, Ariyanon W et al (2013) Cardiac surgery-associated acute kidney injury. Cardiorenal Med 3(3):178–199
14. Zangrillo A, Biondi-Zoccai GG, Frati E et al (2012) Fenoldopam and acute renal failure in cardiac surgery: a meta-analysis of randomized placebo-controlled trials. J Cardiothorac Vasc Anesth 26(3):407–413
15. Bellomo R, Ronco C, Kellum JA et al (2004) Acute renal failure – definition, outcome measures, animal models, fluid therapy and information technology needs: the second international consensus conference of the Acute Dialysis Quality Initiative (ADQI) group. Crit Care 8:R204–R212
16. Legrand M, Darmon M, Joannidis M (2015) Fenoldopam and acute kidney injury. JAMA 313(9):970–971
17. Bove T, Landoni G, Calabrò MG et al (2005) Renoprotective action of fenoldopam in high-risk patients undergoing cardiac surgery: a prospective, double-blind, randomized clinical trial. Circulation 111(24):3230–3235
18. Meco M, Cirri S (2010) The effect of various fenoldopam doses on renal perfusion in patients undergoing cardiac surgery. Ann Thorac Surg 89(2):497–503
19. Choi MR, Kouyoumdzian NM, Rukavina Mikusic NL et al (2015) Renal dopaminergic system: pathophysiological implications and clinical perspectives. World J Nephrol 4(2):196–212
20. Varon J, Marik PE (2003) Clinical review: the management of hypertensive crises. Crit Care 7(5):374–384
21. Parolari A, Pesce LL, Pacini D et al (2012) Risk factors for perioperative acute kidney injury after adult cardiac surgery: role of perioperative management. Ann Thorac Surg 93(2):584–591
22. Bagshaw SM, George C, Bellomo R (2008) Early acute kidney injury and sepsis: a multicentre evaluation. Crit Care 12:R47
23. Glodowski SD, Wagener G (2015) New insights into the mechanisms of acute kidney injury in the intensive care unit. J Clin Anesth 27:175–180
24. Ishimoto Y, Inagi R (2015) Mitochondria: a therapeutic target in acute kidney injury. Nephrol Dial Transplant. pii: gfv317 [Epub ahead of print]
25. Tábara LC, Poveda J, Martin-Cleary C et al (2014) Mitochondria-targeted therapies for acute kidney injury. Expert Rev Mol Med 16:e13

Vasopressin to Reduce Mortality in Patients with Septic Shock and Acute Kidney Injury

14

Linsey E. Christie and Michelle A. Hayes

14.1 General Principles

14.1.1 What Is Vasopressin?

The nonapeptide vasopressin (antidiuretic hormone (ADH)) is synthesized as a prohormone in the magnocellular neurons of the hypothalamic paraventricular and supraoptic nuclei and released from the posterior pituitary. It has a normal plasma concentration of <4 pg/mL and a half-life of 10–35 min [1–3].

14.1.2 How Does Vasopressin Work?

Physiologically, vasopressin mainly controls osmolarity. By stimulation of vasopressin type 2 receptors (V_2Rs) in the renal distal convoluted tubule, it enhances water reabsorption, which causes osmolarity to fall. In shock, vasopressin increases blood pressure by acting on vascular smooth muscle vasopressin type 1 receptors (V_1Rs), causing vasoconstriction [1]. Vasopressin weakly vasoconstricts normal subjects who have an intact autonomic nervous system, as it resets the cardiac baroreflex to a lower pressure. Therefore, very high vasopressin levels (>100 pg/mL) are required to increase mean arterial pressure (MAP) [3, 4]. Vasopressin acts on three types of vasopressin receptors (V_1R, V_2R, and V_3R) as well as on oxytocin-type receptors (OTRs) [2, 3]:

L.E. Christie, MBChB, BSc(Hons), MRCP, FRCA, FHEA, FFICM
M.A. Hayes, MD, FRCA, FFICM (✉)
Magill Department of Anaesthesia and Intensive Care, Chelsea and Westminster Hospital, 369 Fulham Road, London SW10 9NH, UK
e-mail: linsey.christie@nhs.net; michelle.hayes@chelwest.nhs.uk

© Springer International Publishing Switzerland 2016

G. Landoni et al. (eds.), *Reducing Mortality in Acute Kidney Injury*,
DOI 10.1007/978-3-319-33429-5_14

- V_1Rs are found on vascular smooth muscle (systemic, splanchnic, renal, and coronary circulations), myometrium, and platelets. Activation of phospholipase C via Gq G-protein coupled receptors (GPCR) increases intracellular calcium, causing vasoconstriction.
- V_2Rs are present in renal distal convoluted tubules and collecting ducts and on endothelial cells. Activation of adenylate cyclase via Gs-GPCR increases cyclic adenosine 3′,5′-monophosphate (cAMP), leading to aquaporin channel mobilization.
- V_3Rs are mainly found in the pituitary. Phospholipase C activation via Gq-GPCR increases intracellular calcium and releases adrenocorticotrophic hormone (ACTH). Vasopressin may also affect memory and body temperature via V_3Rs.
- OTRs are located in pulmonary, coronary, and cerebral circulatory endothelial cells. Activation results in a calcium-dependent vasodilatory response via nitric oxide.

Vasopressin is used clinically to treat cranial diabetes insipidus, variceal hemorrhage, asystolic cardiac arrest, and septic shock. It is also used to treat von Willebrand's disease (by increasing FVIIIc and von Willebrand factor) and other conditions associated with impaired platelet function (e.g. aspirin use or renal failure) [2, 3].

14.1.3 What Small Studies Have Assessed Vasopressin in Relation to Septic Shock and Acute Kidney Injury?

In 1997, Landry et al. [5] published a case series showing significant increases in urine output in three of five patients receiving vasopressin for septic shock. A later, larger case series demonstrated that in those patients who received vasopressin for septic shock, MAP increased by 18 % at 4 h and remained stable for up to 48 h. Urine output increased by 79 % at 4 h and the mean dose of vasoconstrictor decreased by up to 53 % in the first 48-h period [6].

In 2002, a double-blind randomized controlled trial (RCT) of 24 patients receiving high-dose noradrenaline for septic shock was published [7]. In this study, patients received a 4-h infusion of either noradrenaline or vasopressin. Noradrenaline requirements fell by a greater extent in the vasopressin group at 4 h (median noradrenaline 25–5.3 μg/min compared with 20–17 μg/min). The vasopressin group demonstrated an increased urine output at 4 h (median 32.5–65 mL/h) compared with no change in the noradrenaline group (25–15 mL/h).

In 2006, a small RCT of 23 patients [8] confirmed earlier study findings. In patients with early (<12 h) hyperdynamic, septic shock, vasopressin (dose 0.04–0.2 U/min, $n=13$) was compared with noradrenaline (dose 0.1–2.8 μg kg^{-1} min^{-1}, $n=10$) used to target a MAP ≥70 mmHg for 48 h. Compared to baseline, the vasopressin group had increased systemic vascular resistance (SVR), decreased noradrenaline requirement, decreased cardiac output (decreased heart rate), increased creatinine clearance, and reduced sequential organ failure assessment (SOFA) scores.

In summary, these small studies demonstrate that vasopressin increases MAP, glomerular filtration rate (GFR), urine output, and creatinine clearance; therefore, vasopressin appears to have a beneficial effect in septic shock.

14.1.4 VASST Trial

Russell and colleagues published the Vasopressin and Septic Shock Trial (VASST) [9] in 2008. This was a multicenter double-blind RCT of 778 adult patients receiving a minimum of 5 μg/min noradrenaline. Patients were randomized to either a blinded infusion of vasopressin (0.01–0.03 units/min) or noradrenaline (5–15 μg/min). Other pressor agents could be titrated if target MAP was not being met by infusion of the study drug. Low-dose vasopressin had no effect on the primary outcome of 28-day all-cause mortality. However, in the predefined group of less severe shock, the 28-day mortality rate was significantly lower in the vasopressin group than the noradrenaline group (26.5 % vs. 35.7 %, $p = 0.05$).

14.2 Main Evidence

The main studies evaluating the role of vasopressin on mortality are summarized below.

14.2.1 Gordon (2010) [10]

Key Point Vasopressin may reduce progression to renal failure and mortality in septic shock patients at risk for acute kidney injury (AKI).

In this post hoc analysis of the VASST [9], RIFLE criteria (see Chap. 2) were used to compare vasopressin and noradrenaline. At study entry, 464 patients (59.6 %) had AKI. In the "Risk" category (106 patients), vasopressin use was associated with a lower rate of progression to renal "Failure" or "Loss" categories than noradrenaline (20.8 % vs. 39.6 %, $p = 0.03$). Vasopressin use was associated with both a lower rate of renal replacement therapy (17 % vs. 37.7 %, $p = 0.02$) and a trend to reduced creatinine over the 28-day study period. Mortality rates in the "Risk" category patients were lower in those treated with vasopressin (30.8 % vs. 54.7 %, $p = 0.01$), but this did not reach significance in a multiple logistic regression analysis [10].

There were a number of study limitations. The incidence of AKI may have been underestimated, as they were unable to assess the urine output criteria of the RIFLE definition. It is also not clear whether the benefits seen were due specifically to noradrenaline dose reduction. Furthermore, the number of patients in each RIFLE category was small and differences seen may have been due to chance.

14.2.2 Gordon (2015) [11]

Key Point Vasopressin may reduce use of renal replacement therapy in patients with septic shock, but it does not affect the number of renal failure-free days or mortality.

Following the VASST, VANISH was designed and the protocol published [12]. The preliminary results have been presented at the 2015 ESICM conference. It was a factorial 2×2 design, double-blind RCT. Patients with septic shock were randomized within 6 h to vasopressin (0–0.06 units/min) or noradrenaline (0–12 μg/min) and either hydrocortisone (50 mg intravenously four times daily) or placebo (0.5 mL 0.9 % NaCl). 2,213 patients were screened and 414 were randomized and included. The primary outcome of the trial was the number of renal failure-free days. Comparing all patients in each group, the renal failure-free days were 19 (±11) in the vasopressin group and 20 (±11) in the noradrenaline group [mean (±SD)]. Regarding RRT, 25.5 % of patients required RRT in the vasopressin group and 35.3 % in the noradrenaline group (an absolute difference of −9.8 %, 95 % CI −18.8 to −1.6). The 28-day mortality in the vasopressin group was 30.9 % compared with 27.5 % in the noradrenaline group (an absolute difference of 3.4 %, 95 % CI −5.4 to 12.2).

14.2.3 Kiser (2005) [13]

Key Point Vasopressin may have mortality benefits in treating patients with hepatorenal syndrome (HRS), when compared with octreotide.

Kiser et al. [13] performed a single-center observational study (January 2000 to December 2003) of 43 patients with HRS receiving octreotide, vasopressin, or both. Patients treated with vasopressin alone or in combination with octreotide had significantly greater recovery than those receiving octreotide alone (42 % vs. 38 % vs. 0 %, respectively, $p=0.01$). Patients who responded to therapy had improved mortality (23 % vs. 67 %, $p=0.008$) and were more likely to receive a liver transplant (23 % vs. 0 %, $p=0.005$).

14.3 Pharmacologic Properties: Why Might Vasopressin Benefit Mortality in Patients with Septic Shock and AKI?

The rationale is based upon its pharmacological actions and the pathophysiology of septic shock. Vasopressin potentially increases GFR and renal perfusion more than noradrenaline. An explanation is that there is a greater distribution of V_1Rs on the renal efferent than afferent arterioles. Accordingly, vasopressin constricts the efferent more than the afferent arterioles, thus increasing GFR, unlike noradrenaline which vasoconstricts both [1].

In septic shock, plasma vasopressin levels firstly transiently rise. Subsequently, for unknown reasons, there is a relative vasopressin deficiency, in contrast to other types of shock [1, 3]. Postulated mechanisms include pituitary depletion of vasopressin following the initial surge, autonomic dysfunction in septic shock patients, and increased nitric oxide within the posterior pituitary vascular endothelium, which downregulates vasopressin production [3]. Septic shock also causes hypersensitivity to exogenous vasopressin [1, 3].

14.4 Therapeutic Use

14.4.1 Pharmacokinetics

Vasopressin is a clear, colorless solution stored in a glass vial (2–8 °C). It is rapidly metabolized by liver and kidney vasopressinases, with a half-life of 10–35 min [3].

14.4.2 Dosage/Practical Application

The maximum dose administered in the VASST study was 0.03 U/min [9]. A retrospective case series suggested that higher doses of vasopressin (>0.05 U/min) were associated with increased rates of cardiac arrest [1]. However, a recent prospective study found no adverse effects at 0.067 U/min [12]. Much higher doses (mean 0.23 U/min) were used in a study of hepatorenal syndrome with no difference in the rate of adverse events when compared with noradrenaline [14]. In practice, vasopressin is currently administered for septic shock at 0.01–0.03 U/min via a central venous line. Usually, 20 units are diluted in 50 mL 0.9 % sodium chloride. While vasopressin demonstrates promise in patients with septic shock and AKI, it should not be used routinely with the intent to increase survival [15].

14.4.3 Contraindications (Manufacturer's Instructions)

- Allergy to vasopressin or ingredients
- Chronic nephritis
- Coronary artery disease
- Combination with halogenated anesthetic agents

14.4.4 Adverse Effects

A predictable side effect of vasopressin is water intoxication and hyponatremia given its use in diabetes insipidus. It also decreases cardiac output (by a reduction in heart rate) and may cause myocardial ischemia [1]. Gastrointestinal side effects can occur, ranging from nausea and vomiting to mild abdominal pain and bloating.

There is contradictory evidence as to whether it causes mesenteric ischemia, although its beneficial effect in bleeding esophageal varices is due to splanchnic hypoperfusion. Vasopressin use can also lead to deranged liver function. The hematological side effects include reduced platelet counts and platelet aggregation. The latter can lead to ischemic skin lesions. There is also the potential for extravasation-related skin necrosis and allergies in response to administration.

However, in the VASST study (in which 396 patients received vasopressin), there were no safety concerns [9]. The overall serious adverse event rate was 10.3 % in the vasopressin group and 10.5 % in the noradrenaline group, with no differences in event types.

14.4.5 Timing

Whether vasopressin should be given earlier in the disease process, with more reversible pathology, is the subject of the recently presented VANISH (*va*sopressin versus *n*oradrenaline as the *i*nitial therapy in *s*eptic s*h*ock) UK trial [11, 12]. VANISH, a multicenter double-blind factorial RCT in adults with septic shock, had two primary aims:

1. To determine if vasopressin reduces renal dysfunction compared to noradrenaline when used as the initial vasopressor (see Sect. 14.2.2)
2. To determine any interaction between vasopressin and corticosteroids (see below)

14.4.6 Synergism and Antagonism

The antidiuretic action of vasopressin can be potentiated by carbamazepine, chlorpropamide, clofibrate, urea, fludrocortisones, and tricyclic antidepressants. Conversely, demeclocycline, noradrenaline, lithium, heparin, and alcohol may decrease the antidiuretic action of vasopressin. Ganglionic blockers may increase sensitivity to vasopressin's vasoconstrictor effect. QT interval prolongation is a risk when vasopressin is associated to dolasetron. Vasopressin enhances the sensitivity of the vasculature to other vasopressors.

Of particular interest is that, corticosteroids may interact with vasopressin [16, 17]. In 2014, Gordon et al. [18] demonstrated in a multicenter prospective pilot RCT of 61 patients with septic shock that coadministration of hydrocortisone and vasopressin reduced vasopressin requirements (dose and duration) but not plasma vasopressin levels. The interaction between vasopressin and corticosteroids has been investigated further in the VANISH trial [11, 12]. This study showed that the combination of noradrenaline or vasopressin with hydrocortisone had no effect on 28-day mortality in patients with septic shock.

Clinical Summary

Drug	Indications	Cautions	Side effects	Dose	Notes
Vasopressin	Septic shock and AKI	Heart failure or any condition exacerbated by fluid retention Hypertension or any condition exacerbated by hypertension Lactation, pregnancy	Decreased cardiac output Myocardial ischemia Mesenteric ischemia (unclear) Reduced platelet count Skin necrosis (extravasation)	0.01–0.03 U/min for septic shock May be safe to use higher doses but lack of evidence currently	Septic shock causes: 1. Initial surge then relative deficiency of vasopressin 2. Hypersensitivity to exogenous vasopressin Exact role and timing of vasopressin are unclear (the VANISH trial is in progress and may add new insights)

References

1. Gordon AC (2011) Vasopressin in septic shock. J Intensive Care Soc 12:11–14
2. Sharman A, Low J (2008) Vasopressin and its role in critical care. Contin Educ Anaesth Crit Care Pain 8:134–137
3. Holmes CL, Patel BM, Russell JA, Walley KR (2001) Physiology of vasopressin relevant to management of septic shock. Chest 120:989–1002
4. Mohring J, Glanzer K, Maciel JA Jr et al (1980) Greatly enhanced pressor response to antidiuretic hormone in patients with impaired cardiovascular reflexes due to idiopathic orthostatic hypotension. J Cardiovasc Pharmacol 2:367–376
5. Landry DW, Levin HR, Gallant EM et al (1997) Vasopressin pressor hypersensitivity in vasodilatory septic shock. Crit Care Med 27:1416–1421
6. Holmes CL, Walley KR, Chittock DR et al (2001) The effects of vasopressin on hemodynamics and renal function in severe septic shock: a case series. Intensive Care Med 27: 1416–1421
7. Patel BM, Chittock DR, Russell JA, Walley KR (2002) Beneficial effects of short-term vasopressin infusion during severe septic shock. Anesthesiology 96:576–582
8. Lauzier F, Levy B, Lamarre P et al (2006) Vasopressin or norepinephrine in early haemodynamic septic shock: a randomized clinical trial. Intensive Care Med 32:1783–1789
9. Russell JA, Walley KR, Singer J et al (2008) Vasopressin versus norepinephrine infusion in patients with septic shock. N Engl J Med 358:877–887
10. Gordon AC, Russell JA, Walley KR et al (2010) The effects of vasopressin on acute kidney injury in septic shock. Intensive Care Med 36:83–91
11. Gordon AC et al (2015) Vasopressin vs Noradrenaline as Initial Therapy in Septic Shock (VANISH): a randomized controlled trial. In: *Hot topics session.* Symposium conducted at the European Society for Intensive Care Medicine (ESICM) lives 2015 conference, Berlin

12. Gordon AC, Mason AJ, Perkins GD et al (2014) Protocol for a randomised controlled trial of VAsopressin versus Noradrenaline as Initial therapy in Septic sHock (VANISH). BMJ Open 4:e005866
13. Kiser TH, Fish DN, Obritsch MD et al (2005) Vasopressin, not octreotide, may be beneficial in the treatment of hepatorenal syndrome: a retrospective study. Nephrol Dial Transplant 20:1813–1820
14. Torgersen C, Dunser MW, Wenzel V et al (2010) Comparing two different arginine vasopressin doses in advanced vasodilatory shock: a randomized, controlled, open label trial. Intensive Care Med 36:57–65
15. Landoni G, Bove T, Székely A et al (2013) Reducing mortality in acute kidney injury patients: systematic review and international web-based survey. J Cardiothorac Vasc Anesth 27:1384–1398
16. Russell JA, Walley KR, Gordon AC et al (2009) Interaction of vasopressin infusion, corticosteroid treatment, and mortality of septic shock. Crit Care 37:811–818
17. Annane D (2009) Vasopressin plus corticosteroids: the shock duo! Crit Care Med 37:1126–1127
18. Gordon AC, Mason AJ, Perkins GD et al (2014) The interaction of vasopressin and corticosteroids in septic shock: a pilot randomized controlled trial. Crit Care Med 42:1325–1333

Terlipressin Reduces Mortality in Hepatorenal Syndrome

15

Rakhi Maiwall and Shiv Kumar Sarin

15.1 General Principles

Type 1 hepatorenal syndrome (HRS) is a severe complication of cirrhosis, which is associated with an unacceptably high mortality rate of 80 % at 2 weeks if untreated [1]. It was previously defined as a rapidly progressive decline in renal function, characterized by doubling of the initial creatinine to a level of more than 2.5 mg/dL in 2 weeks. Severe circulatory dysfunction, along with an inadequate cardiac contractility as a manifestation of cirrhosis-related cardiomyopathy, has been reported as the pathophysiologic hallmark of HRS [1]. Several studies have shown that an adequate mean arterial pressure (MAP) is pivotal for HRS reversal, in order to counteract the exaggerated systemic vasodilation state. Accordingly, the administration of vasoconstrictors (along with albumin) is recommended in patients with HRS (See Chap. 16, Fig. 16.1). A good long-term survival has been reported for HRS after orthotopic liver transplantation (OLT) [1]. However, reversal with medical therapy remains of the utmost importance. The association of terlipressin and albumin has been shown to be an effective treatment for type 1 HRS, and both transplant-free survival and survival after OLT are strongly related to the improvement of renal function after this treatment [1].

Various classes of vasoconstrictors have the potential to reverse HRS, including vasopressin analogues (terlipressin and ornipressin), alpha-1 adrenergic receptor agonists (midodrine and norepinephrine), and somatostatin analogues (octreotide). This chapter will focus on the use of terlipressin for the treatment of HRS, with particular focus on its impact on mortality.

R. Maiwall • S.K. Sarin, DM, FNA, DSc (Hon). (✉)
Department of Hepatology, Institute of Liver and Biliary Sciences,
D-1, Vasant Kunj, New Delhi 110070, India
e-mail: rakhi_2011@yahoo.co.in; sksarin@ilbs.in

© Springer International Publishing Switzerland 2016

G. Landoni et al. (eds.), *Reducing Mortality in Acute Kidney Injury*,
DOI 10.1007/978-3-319-33429-5_15

15.2 Main Evidence

To date, various trials have assessed the efficacy of terlipressin in the reversal of HRS. The majority of them have used terlipressin in combination with albumin, while others have compared its efficacy against other vasoconstrictors (Table 15.1).

15.2.1 Terlipressin Without Albumin Versus Placebo

In the initial randomized controlled trial (RCT) by Solanki et al. [2], terlipressin administration was shown to result in significant improvement in urine output, creatinine clearance, serum creatinine, MAP, and survival as compared to placebo. Subsequently, in a series of 69 patients, Testro et al. [3] reported reversal of HRS type 1 in 41 patients (59.4 %) and improvement in survival in 21 (30.4 %).

15.2.2 Terlipressin with Albumin vs. Placebo

In a prospective RCT, Sanyal and colleagues [4] showed the superiority of terlipressin (in association with albumin) over placebo in HRS reversal, which translated into improved survival at 6 months. A significant improvement in renal function with terlipressin and albumin, as compared to placebo, was also found in the RCT by Martin Llahi et al. [5], but without any difference in 3-month survival between the two groups. Finally, consistent with the findings of Sanyal and colleagues [4], Neri et al. [6] showed a significant improvement in both renal function and survival in patients receiving terlipressin plus albumin.

15.2.3 Terlipressin and Meta-analyses

Sagi et al. [7] analyzed data from four RCTs (including a total of 223 patients) and showed that terlipressin is effective in reversing type 1 HRS and improving survival. The meta-analysis by Fabrizi et al. [8] consistently demonstrated that discontinuation of therapy with terlipressin was significantly associated with an increase in the number of relapses [8]. However, even though terlipressin improved HRS reversal, it did not impact overall survival. Conversely, a Cochrane systematic review of ten RCTs investigating the effects of vasoconstrictors in the treatment of HRS suggested a reduced mortality with terlipressin [9]. In fact, in the six studies reporting data on mortality, a total of 155 subjects were randomized to receive terlipressin, either alone or with albumin (74 patients), or no intervention as either placebo or albumin (98 patients). Subanalysis using random effects model found that terlipressin administration was associated with reduced mortality (relative risk [RR] 0.80, 95 % confidence interval [CI] 0.66–0.97). Yet, all studies had high risk of bias.

Table 15.1 Summary of clinical trials evaluating the therapeutic efficacy of terlipressin

References	*N*	Study design	End points	Dose and route	Results	Safety
Solanki et al. (2003) [2]	Total 24 Terlipressin 12 (Gp A) Placebo 12 (Gp B)	Randomized controlled single-blinded trial	Reversal of HRS survival at 15 days	1 mg i.v. q 12 h placebo q 12 h	Serum creatinine decreased in Gp A as compared to Gp B ($p<0.05$) Mean arterial pressure increased significantly ($p<0.05$) in Gp A Survival: 5 patients in Gp A compared with none in Gp B at day 15 ($p<0.05$)	Transient self-limiting side effects; crampy abdominal pain (2 patients) Cardiac arrhythmias (3 patients)
Sanyal et al. (2008) [4]	Total 112 Terlipressin + albumin 56 Placebo + albumin 56	Randomized, double-blind, placebo-controlled trial	Decrease in SCr level to ≤1.5 mg/dL for at least 48 h by day 14 without dialysis, death, or relapse of HRS type 1	1 mg i.v. q 6 h dose was doubled on day 4 if serum creatinine did not decrease by 30 % of baseline	Improvement in serum creatinine and HRS reversal better with terlipressin as compared to placebo (–0.7 mg/dL; $p<0.009$ and $p=0.008$, 34 % vs. 13 %, respectively)	Total adverse event rate similar to placebo Nonfatal myocardial infarction (1 patient)

(continued)

Table 15.1 (continued)

References	*N*	Study design	End points	Dose and route	Results	Safety
Martin Llahi et al. (2008) [5]	Total 46 Terlipressin + albumin 23 Albumin alone 23	Randomized controlled trial	Improvement of renal function and survival at 3 months	Terlipressin 1–2 mg/4 h i.v. and albumin 1 g/kg followed by 20–40 g/day	Improvement of renal functions (43.5 % vs. 8.7 %, $p=0.017$) No difference in survival at 3 months (27 % vs. 19 %, $p=0.7$)	Cardiovascular complications (10 patients in terlipressin Gp vs. 4 patients in albumin Gp) Terlipressin withdrawal (3 cases)
Neri et al. (2008) [6]	Total 52 Terlipressin + albumin 26 Albumin 26	Controlled trial	Improvement in liver and renal function, plasma renin activity, and aldosterone		Significant improvement in renal function ($p<0.001$) and survival ($p<0.0001$) in terlipressin Gp as compared to albumin-only Gp	–
Alessandria et al. (2007) [10]	Total 22 HRS type 1 (9) HRS type 2 (13)	Randomized controlled trial	Assessing the efficacy and safety of noradrenaline vs. terlipressin in patients with HRS	Noradrenaline (0.1–0.7 μg/kg/min) and albumin (10 patients) or terlipressin (1–2 mg/4 h) and albumin (12 patients)	Reversal of HRS 70 % of patients treated with noradrenaline and 83 % of patients treated with terlipressin, p = n.s.	No patient developed signs of myocardial ischemia

Cavallin et al. (2015) [13]	Total 49 Terlipressin + albumin 27 Octreotide/M Midodrine + albumin 22	Randomized controlled trial	To compare the effectiveness of terlipressin plus albumin vs. midodrine and octreotide plus albumin in the treatment of HRS	Terlipressin i.v. infusion, 3 mg/24 h, increased to 12 mg/24 h based on response. Midodrine orally at an initial dose of 7.5 mg thrice daily to a maximum of 12.5 mg thrice daily. Octreotide 100 μg subcutaneous thrice daily up to 200 μg thrice daily Albumin 1 g/kg on day 1 and 20–40 g/day thereafter	Recovery of renal function is significantly better in terlipressin (19/27, 70.4 %) compared to the midodrine-octreotide group (6/21, 28.6 %) ($p = 0.01$). Improvement in renal function and lower baseline MELD score were associated with better survival	

(continued)

Table 15.1 (continued)

References	*N*	Study design	End points	Dose and route	Results	Safety
Sharma et al. (2008) [11]	Total 40 Gp A (noradrenaline + albumin) 20 Gp B (terlipressin + albumin) 20	Open-label, randomized, pilot trial	To assess the efficacy of terlipressin and noradrenaline on renal function and clinical outcome of patients with HRS type 1 and assess predictors of response	Noradrenaline 0.5–3.0 mg/h Terlipressin 0.5–2 mg i.v. q 6 hourly	Reversal of HRS was similar in both groups: 10 patients (50 %) in both groups had a significant ($p<0.05$) decrease in serum creatinine from baseline MAP and urine output significantly increased in both groups with therapy 11 patients (55 %) in Gp A and a similar number in Gp B survived until day 15 ($p=0.798$)	Reversible cardiac ischemia in one patient in each group

Gp group, *MELD* model for end-stage liver disease, *n.s.* not significant

15.2.4 Terlipressin vs. Other Vasoconstrictors

- *Terlipressin vs. Noradrenaline.* An unblinded pilot investigation on cirrhotic patients with HRS suggested that noradrenaline was as effective and safe as terlipressin [10]. Following this, Sharma et al. [11] showed an improvement in both renal function and survival with noradrenaline, as compared to terlipressin, in an open-label RCT. Interestingly, in a recent meta-analysis including four studies (154 patients, overall), no difference in reversal of HRS (RR0.97, 95 % CI0.76–1.23), 1-month mortality (RR0.89, 95 % CI0.68–1.17), and recurrence of HRS (RR0.72, 95 % CI0.36–1.45) was noted between norepinephrine and terlipressin [12], although adverse events were less frequent with noradrenaline. However, all trials were at high risk of bias.
- *Terlipressin vs. Octreotide and Midodrine.* In an RCT, a significantly higher rate of recovery of renal function was found with terlipressin (19/27, 70.4 %) as compared to octreotide and midodrine (6/21, 28.6 %) [13]. The trial had to be stopped early after an interim analysis reported a superiority of the intervention (terlipressin) in comparison to standard therapy (midodrine plus octreotide). Importantly, terlipressin was administered as a continuous infusion, which may have accounted for the superior rate of HRS reversal noted in this trial.

15.2.5 Predictors of Response to Terlipressin

Various predictors have been identified for a non-response to terlipressin treatment, including high baseline value of serum creatinine and total serum bilirubin, failure to increase MAP and cardiac output, and the presence of underlying tubular dysfunction [14]. Among these factors, identifying significant values of high serum creatinine is of particular clinical importance. In fact, serum creatinine is known to underestimate the severity of renal dysfunction in patients with cirrhosis as it can be spuriously recorded as low. This occurs in the presence of marked hyperbilirubinemia, hemolysis, decreased creatine synthesis, reduced muscle mass, and increased renal tubular creatinine secretion. In order to diagnose HRS early and remove reliance on serum creatinine, the revised criteria for HRS (HRS-AKI) were proposed by the International Club of Ascites (ICA) in 2015 (Fig. 15.1) [15]. This is wherein an absolute cutoff for serum creatinine has been removed. Rodriguez et al. [16] recently evaluated patients with HRS associated with bacterial infections, in which poor response to terlipressin was directly related to the severity of liver failure and to the non-resolution of infection. A strong interaction was noted between the resolution of bacterial infection, as well as severity of liver failure, and extrahepatic organ failure. Similarly, we have also reported a lower response to terlipressin in patients with acute-on-chronic liver failure (ACLF) [17]. However, it is still unclear if the poor response

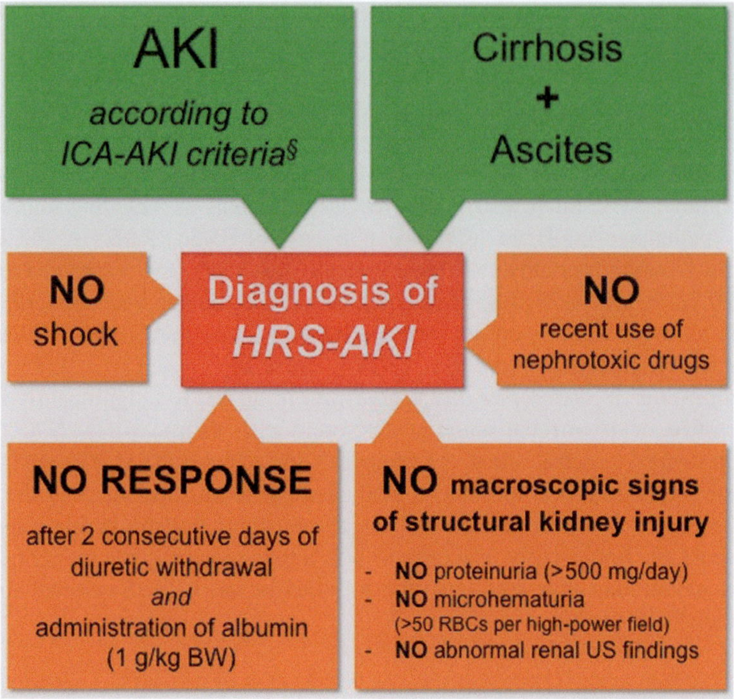

Fig. 15.1 Diagnostic criteria for hepatorenal syndrome type of acute kidney injury (HRS-AKI) in patients with cirrhosis proposed by the International Club of Ascites (ICA) [15]. ICA-AKI, International Club of Ascites-Acute Kidney Injury; BW, body weight; RBCs, red blood cells; US, ultrasonography. §See Chapter 16, Table 16.1

to terlipressin in ACLF patients is associated with a progression to acute tubular necrosis, an inadequate cardiac output secondary to bacterial infection, the severity of systemic inflammation, or a different pathophysiologic basis of kidney injury in these patients [16, 17].

15.3 Pathophysiologic Principles/Pharmacologic Properties

HRS is characterized by profound circulatory dysfunction. The main mediators are nitric oxide (NO) and carbon monoxide, which together cause marked splanchnic and systemic arterial vasodilation and a reduction in the effective arterial blood volume. Nitric oxide also causes negative inotropic effects via increased cyclic guanosine monophosphate (cGMP) production, leading to cardiac dysfunction. This in turn causes activation of the renin-angiotensin-aldosterone systems (RAAS) as well as an intense renal vasoconstriction with a consequent decrease in renal blood flow.

It has also been shown that any factor that worsens the vasodilatory state or decreases blood volume can further perturb renal perfusion and lead to renal dysfunction [1]. Moreover, it has been shown that patients with bacterial infections have an increased severity of cardiac and renal dysfunction secondary to an exaggerated systemic inflammatory response with increased levels of pro-inflammatory cytokines (such as TNFα and IL-6).

Terlipressin is a prohormone of lysine vasopressin (triglycyl lysine vasopressin). The glycyl residues are cleaved by endothelial peptidases after intravenous administration, enabling prolonged release of lysine vasopressin. Terlipressin has an affinity for both V_1 and V_2 receptors (see Chap. 14). V_1 receptor stimulation causes splanchnic vasoconstriction and, accordingly, reduction in splanchnic blood flow and portal pressure, leading to the amelioration of the hyperdynamic circulation, thereby improving the effective circulatory volume and renal perfusion pressure (Fig. 15.2). Additionally, V_2 receptor stimulation by terlipressin increases water reabsorption in the renal collecting ducts by mobilizing the expression of aquaporin-2 water channels in the apical plasma membrane [18].

15.4 Therapeutic Use

Terlipressin is usually administered at a dose of 0.5–1 mg intravenously every 4–6 h (4–6 mg/day). The dose can be increased up to 2 mg every 4 h if baseline serum creatinine level does not improve by 25 % at day 3 of therapy. Alternatively, terlipressin can be administered as continuous intravenous infusion [18, 19]. The treatment should be continued until resolution of AKI. Adverse events, mainly including ischemic events involving the heart, fingers, and mesenteries, are reported in approximately 5–12 % of patients during terlipressin treatment. There is evidence that when terlipressin is administered using continuous infusion rather than as a bolus for the treatment of HRS, better efficacy can be achieved with a lower total daily dose and with fewer side effects [13, 19].

15.5 Future Perspectives

There is emerging data suggesting the presence of structural renal damages in patients with cirrhosis and a presumed diagnosis of HRS [17]. Moreover, patients with ACLF develop structural kidney damage more often as compared to patients with cirrhosis [17]. RCTs are therefore needed in order to assess the efficacy of terlipressin as compared to other vasoconstrictors specifically in patients with ACLF, as well as to identify the frequency and predictors of non-response to the drug. Two other groups where terlipressin needs to be studied, which are

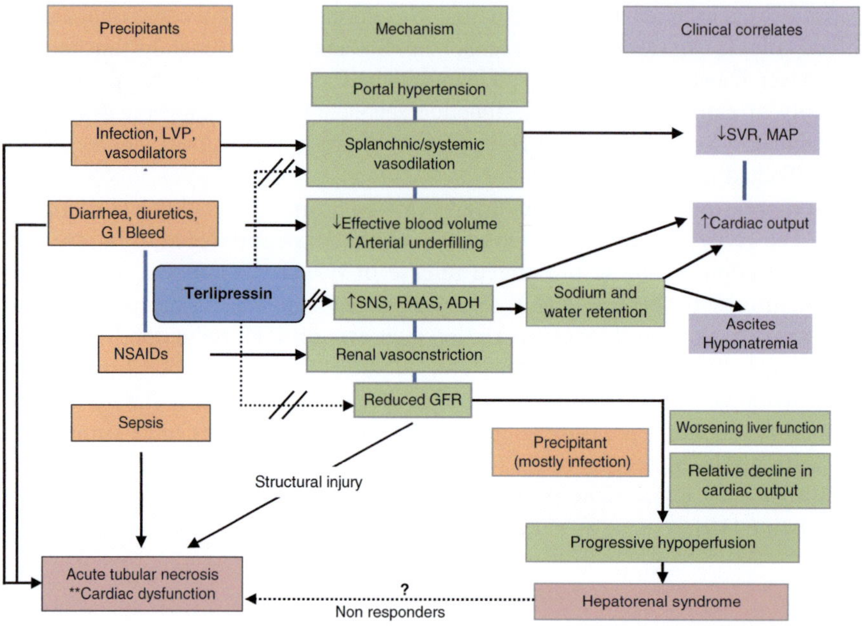

Fig. 15.2 Pathophysiology of hepatorenal syndrome (*HRS*) and role of terlipressin. In patients with cirrhosis, portal hypertension causes splanchnic and systemic vasodilatation, decreasing the effective arterial blood volume. The consequent activation of sympathetic nervous system (*SNS*), renin-angiotensin-aldosterone system (*RAAS*), and antidiuretic hormone (*ADH*) leads to retention of sodium and water, formation of ascites, dilutional hyponatremia, and decrease in systemic vascular resistances (*SVR*) and mean arterial pressure (*MAP*). At the same time, chronic renal vasoconstriction and decreased renal perfusion occur. Factors disrupting the resulting precarious balance, such as nonsteroidal anti-inflammatory drugs (*NSAIDs*), vasodilators, infections, large-volume paracentesis (*LVP*), gastrointestinal (*GI*) bleed, diarrhea, and excessive diuresis due to diuretics, may precipitate AKI. Cirrhotic cardiomyopathy is often associated. Vasoconstrictors such as terlipressin are effective in reversing HRS in 30–50 % of patients by acting at various levels (*double-slashed arrows*). Possible mechanisms of non-response are presence of structural tubular injury, failure to increase cardiac output, severity of liver failure, and inflammation-associated renal dysfunction (*dashed lines*)

currently excluded from the diagnostic criteria for HRS, include patients with cirrhosis with acute-on-chronic kidney disease, in which vasoconstrictors may reverse the acute component, and patients with cirrhosis and septic shock. Preliminary data from our group has reported the efficacy of terlipressin against noradrenaline in improving renal function in cirrhotic patients with septic shock [20]. The management of non-responders still remains an unmet challenge. It is also important to understand the role of dialysis and artificial liver support in ACLF patients with HRS. Lastly, the efficacy of terlipressin in the treatment of HRS needs to be reassessed in future studies considering the revised criteria for HRS-AKI.

Clinical Summary

Drug	Indication	Cautions	Side effects	Dose	Notes
Terlipressin	Hepatorenal syndrome type 1	Ischemic heart disease Known hypersensitivity Chronic kidney disease Pregnancy Mesenteric ischemia Peripheral arterial disease	Cardiac: atrial fibrillation, ventricular extrasystoles, torsade de pointes, tachycardia, myocardial infarction, hypertension Gastrointestinal: abdominal cramps, loose stools, nausea, intestinal ischemia Skin and subcutaneous tissue: peripheral cyanosis and gangrene Others: hyponatremia in patients with variceal bleeding	Starting dose 2 mg daily, possibly increased up to 12 mg/day (as bolus or continuous infusion)	Most common adverse effects (1–10 %) are paleness, hypertension, abdominal pain, nausea, diarrhea, and headache Drug interactions: terlipressin potentiates the hypotensive effect of nonselective beta-blockers on the portal vein Concomitant treatment with drugs with a known bradycardic effect (e.g., propofol, sufentanil) may reduce heart rate and cardiac output and should therefore be avoided

References

1. Gines P, Schrier RW et al (2009) Renal failure in cirrhosis. N Engl J Med 361:1279–1290
2. Solanki P, Chawla A, Garg R et al (2003) Beneficial effects of terlipressin in hepatorenal syndrome: a prospective, randomized placebo-controlled clinical trial. J Gastroenterol Hepatol 18(2):152–156
3. Testro AG, Wongseelashote S, Angus PW et al (2008) Long-term outcome of patients treated with terlipressin for types 1 and 2 hepatorenal syndrome. J Gastroenterol Hepatol 23:1535–1540

4. Sanyal AJ, Boyer T, Garcia-Tsao G et al (2008) A randomized prospective double-blind placebo controlled trail of terlipressin in type 1 Hepatorenal syndrome. Gastroenterology 134:1360–1368
5. Martin Llahi M, Pepin MN, Guavera M et al (2008) Terlipressin plus albumin vs. albumin alone in patients with hepatorenal syndrome: a randomized study. Gastroenterology 134:1352–1359
6. Neri S, Pulvirenti D, Malaguarnera M et al (2008) Terlipressin and albumin in patients with cirrhosis and type I hepatorenal syndrome. Dig Dis Sci 53:830–835
7. Sagi SV, Mittal S, Kasturi KS et al (2010) Terlipressin therapy for reversal of type 1 hepatorenal syndrome: a meta-analysis of randomized controlled trials. J Gastroenterol Hepatol 25:880–885
8. Fabrizi F, Dixit V, Messa P et al (2009) Terlipressin for hepatorenal syndrome: a meta-analysis of randomized trials. Int J Artif Organs 32:133–140
9. Gluud LL, Christensen K, Christensen E et al (2010) Systematic review of randomized trials on vasoconstrictor drugs for hepatorenal syndrome. Hepatology 51:576–584
10. Alessandria C, Ottobrelli A, Debernardi-Venon W et al (2007) Noradrenalin vs. terlipressin in patients with hepatorenal syndrome: a prospective, randomized, unblinded, pilot study. J Hepatol 47:499–505
11. Sharma P, Kumar A, Shrama BC et al (2008) An open label, pilot, randomized controlled trial of noradrenaline versus terlipressin in the treatment of type 1 hepatorenal syndrome and predictors of response. Am J Gastroenterol 103:1689–1697
12. Nassar Junior AP, Farias AQ, D'Albuquerque LA et al (2014) Terlipressin versus norepinephrine in the treatment of hepatorenal syndrome: a systematic review and meta-analysis. PLoS One 9(9):e107466
13. Cavallin M, Kamath PS, Merli M, for the Italian Association for the Study of the Liver Study Group on Hepatorenal Syndrome et al (2015) Terlipressin plus albumin versus midodrine and octreotide plus albumin in the treatment of hepatorenal syndrome: a randomized trial. Hepatology 62(2):567–574
14. Boyer TD, Sanyal AJ, Garcia-Tsao G et al (2011) Terlipressin Study Group. Predictors of response to terlipressin plus albumin in hepatorenal syndrome (HRS) type 1: relationship of serum creatinine to hemodynamics. J Hepatol 55(2):315–321
15. Angeli P, Ginès P, Wong F et al (2015) Diagnosis and management of acute kidney injury in patients with cirrhosis: revised consensus recommendations of the International Club of Ascites. Gut 64(4):531–537
16. Rodríguez E, Elia C, Solà E et al (2014) Terlipressin and albumin for type-1 hepatorenal syndrome associated with sepsis. J Hepatol 60(5):955–961
17. Maiwall R, Sarin SK, Moreau R (2016) Acute kidney injury in acute on chronic liver failure. Hepatol Int 10(2):245–57
18. Sarin SK, Sharma P (2011) Terlipressin: an asset for hepatologists! Hepatology 54(2):724–728
19. Gerbes AL, Huber E, Gülberg V et al (2009) Terlipressin for hepatorenal syndrome: continuous infusion as an alternative to i.v. bolus administration. Gastroenterology 137:1179
20. Choudhury AK, Vashishtha C, Saini D et al (2014) A prospective open label randomized noninferiority trial to compare the efficacy and safety of monotherapy with noradrenaline and terlipressin in patients of cirrhosis with septic shock admitted to the Intensive care unit (NCT01836224). Hepatology 60:254A [Abstract # 113]

Albumin to Reduce Mortality in Cirrhotic Patients with Acute Kidney Injury

16

Christian J. Wiedermann

16.1 General Principles

Acute kidney injury (AKI) occurs in up to one-fifth of cirrhotic patients hospitalized with portal hypertension and portosystemic collaterals [1]. As discussed in Chap. 15 (see Fig. 15.2), these conditions cause systemic and splanchnic vasodilation and, accordingly, a decrease in the "effective" arterial blood volume. As a consequence, antidiuretic hormone (ADH) is released and both renin-angiotensin-aldosterone system (RAAS) and sympathetic nervous system (SNS) are activated, leading to water/sodium retention and, hence, to an increase in intravascular volume. As cirrhosis progresses, these compensatory mechanisms become inadequate, and a further reduction in the effective blood volume leads to pronounced vasoconstriction, involving preferentially renal and central nervous system blood vessels. The consequent reduction in renal blood flow that is typical of advanced cirrhosis is responsible for a decrease in glomerular filtration rate (GFR) and may also contribute to the development of ischemic injury. Even in the presence of low-grade renal hypoperfusion, AKI may develop due to the exposure to nephrotoxic drugs or to conditions causing acute fluctuations in intravascular volume such as gastrointestinal bleeding, diarrhea, use of diuretics, and large-volume (>4–5 L) paracentesis (LVP). The outpatient use of diuretics and the occurrence of lactulose-associated diarrhea are responsible for the majority of AKI cases in cirrhotic patients. Finally, up to 30 % of patients with cirrhosis and ascites develop spontaneous bacterial peritonitis (SBP): in these patients, AKI may also be precipitated by inflammation-associated vasodilation, as well as by the use of potentially nephrotoxic antibiotics prescribed for the treatment of SBP.

C.J. Wiedermann, MD
Department of Internal Medicine, Central Hospital of Bolzano,
Lorenz Böhler Street 5, Bolzano 39100, Italy
e-mail: christian.wiedermann@asbz.it

© Springer International Publishing Switzerland 2016
G. Landoni et al. (eds.), *Reducing Mortality in Acute Kidney Injury*,
DOI 10.1007/978-3-319-33429-5_16

Table 16.1 International Club of Ascites new definitions for the diagnosis and management of acute kidney injury (AKI) in patients with cirrhosis (ICA-AKI)

<table>
<tr><th>Subject</th><th colspan="3">Definition</th></tr>
<tr><td rowspan="2">Baseline sCr</td><td colspan="3">A value of sCr obtained in the previous 3 months, when available, can be used as baseline sCr. In patients with more than one value within the previous 3 months, the value closest to the hospital admission time should be used</td></tr>
<tr><td colspan="3">In patients without a previous sCr value, the sCr on admission should be used as baseline</td></tr>
<tr><td>Definition of AKI</td><td colspan="3">Increase in sCr ≥0.3 mg/dL (≥26.5 μmol/L) within 48 h or a percentage increase sCr ≥50 % from baseline which is known, or presumed, to have occurred within the prior 7 days</td></tr>
<tr><td rowspan="3">Staging of AKI</td><td colspan="3">Stage 1: increase in sCr ≥0.3 mg/dL (26.5 μmol/L) or an increase in sCr ≥1.5-fold to twofold from baseline</td></tr>
<tr><td colspan="3">Stage 2: increase in sCr > two- to threefold from baseline</td></tr>
<tr><td colspan="3">Stage 3: increase of sCr >threefold from baseline or sCr ≥4.0 mg/dL (353.6 μmol/L) with an acute increase ≥0.3 mg/dL (26.5 μmol/L) or initiation of RRT</td></tr>
<tr><td rowspan="2">Progression of AKI</td><td colspan="2">Progression</td><td>Regression</td></tr>
<tr><td colspan="2">Progression of AKI to a higher stage and/or need for RRT</td><td>Regression of AKI to a lower stage</td></tr>
<tr><td rowspan="2">Response to treatment</td><td>No response</td><td>Partial response</td><td>Full response</td></tr>
<tr><td>No regression of AKI</td><td>Regression of AKI stage with a reduction of sCr to ≥0.3 mg/dL (26.5 μmol/L) above the baseline value</td><td>Return of sCr to a value within 0.3 mg/dL (26.5 μmol/L) of the baseline value</td></tr>
</table>

Reproduced with permission from Angeli et al. [1]
RRT renal replacement therapy, *sCr* serum creatinine

AKI is associated with a stepwise increase in the risk of death according to its severity. Since even small increases in serum creatinine (sCr) have been shown to be associated with adverse outcomes, new diagnostic criteria for AKI in cirrhotic patients have been recently introduced that provide higher sensibility for the diagnosis of moderate AKI and allow an earlier identification of severe AKI (Table 16.1) [1].

Although paracentesis is generally the first-line treatment for patients with refractory ascites, it causes further reduction in the effective circulating volume. The consequent pronounced reactivation of RAAS and SNS may be responsible for the so-called post-paracentesis circulatory dysfunction (PPCD), which is associated with a high risk of ascites recurrence, dilutional hyponatremia, development of hepatorenal syndrome (HRS), and death. Unlike prerenal uremia, HRS does not respond to volume expansion [2].

In more than two-thirds of cirrhotic patients, however, AKI is due to renal hypoperfusion and shows an improvement with volume expansion. Administration of human albumin to treat hypovolemia is recommended in cirrhotic patients with AKI [1] and, as discussed below, has been shown to reduce mortality in these patients, especially in those with SBP [3, 4].

16.2 Main Evidence

16.2.1 Albumin, AKI, and Mortality in Cirrhotic Patients

Serum albumin levels have been identified as an independent factor affecting mortality in patients with AKI [5]. Moreover, low serum albumin has been found to be a risk factor for AKI in different clinical settings, including hyperuricemic patients treated with nonsteroidal anti-inflammatory drugs (NSAIDs) [6], patients with cystic fibrosis receiving intravenous aminoglycosides [7], patients with acute coronary syndromes treated with percutaneous coronary intervention (contrast-induced AKI) [8], and surgical patients [9–12]. In particular, preoperative low serum albumin has been shown to be an independent risk factor for AKI following off-pump coronary artery bypass (OPCAB) surgery, which in turn is associated with poor outcomes [9]. Similarly, low serum albumin has been found to be an independent risk factor for postoperative AKI in patients undergoing surgery of the thoracic aorta [10], cardiopulmonary bypass and aortic cross-clamp surgery [11], and esophageal cancer surgery [12]. It is reasonable to expect, therefore, that the administration of albumin would prevent AKI and even reduce mortality in patients with or at risk for AKI.

Moreover, since liberal fluid administration can be associated with AKI and increased mortality in critically ill patients (see also Chap. 19), especially in those with sepsis [13, 14], it has been traditionally believed that the use of colloids (including albumin) for fluid resuscitation could be advantageous in such situations thanks to a reduced risk of overhydration [15]. However, it has been also hypothesized that hyperoncotic colloids might contribute to AKI.

In order to shed some light on this issue, Wiedermann et al. [4] performed a meta-analysis of randomized controlled trials (RCTs) assessing the risk of AKI after infusion of hyperoncotic albumin and hydroxyethyl starch (HES) solutions. Mortality was a secondary end point. Data from 11 RCTs including a total of 1,220 patients were analyzed: 7 studies evaluated hyperoncotic albumin and 4 hyperoncotic HES. Clinical indications for albumin or HES administration were surgery, sepsis, ascites, and SBP, with most studies involving patients with cirrhosis. The risk of AKI was decreased by 76 % with albumin (odds ratio [OR] 0.24, 95 % confidence interval [CI] 0.12–0.48, $p<0.0001$) and increased by 92 % with HES (OR 1.92, 95 % CI 1.31–2.81, $p=0.0008$). Moreover, albumin reduced mortality (OR 0.52, 95 % CI 0.28–0.95, $p=0.035$), while HES increased mortality (OR 1.41, 95 % CI 1.01–1.96, $p=0.043$).

These findings are consistent with those of a previous investigation in which 126 cirrhotic patients with SBP were randomized to receive or not 20 % albumin (at a dose of 1.5 g/kg at the time of diagnosis and 1 g/kg 3 days after) in addition to antibiotic therapy [3]. Nonreversible deterioration of renal function occurred in 10 % of patients receiving antibiotics and albumin as compared with 33 % of patients receiving only antibiotics ($p=0.002$). Furthermore, both in-hospital and 90-day mortality were lower in the albumin group (10 % vs. 29 %, $p=0.01$ and 22 % vs. 41 %, $p=0.03$, respectively).

A trend toward reduced 28-day mortality with albumin was also found in a subgroup analysis of patients with severe sepsis from a large multicenter investigation in which a total of 6,997 intensive care unit (ICU) patients were randomized to receive either 4 % albumin or normal saline for fluid resuscitation (relative risk [RR] 0.87, 95 % CI 0.74–1.02, $p=0.09$) [16].

16.2.2 Albumin and Other Complications of Cirrhosis

There are only a few small studies on the prophylactic effects of albumin against ascites. Lower ascites recurrence and improved survival have been observed in an RCT investigating long-term administration of diuretics plus albumin (25 g per week in the first year and 25 g every 2 weeks thereafter) as compared with diuretics alone [17]. In another study, albumin infusion was as effective as the combination of octreotide and midodrine in preventing ascites recurrence after LVP and was associated with a better outcome [18]. Interestingly, when ascites recurred, sCr levels were lower in the albumin group (0.9 vs. 1.2 mg/dL, $p=0.051$). These effects are thought to be related to the reduced function of endogenous albumin in patients with liver failure [19].

The beneficial effect of albumin infusion on the occurrence of PPCD was first demonstrated in the 1980s [20]. Clinical practice guidelines recommend albumin treatment after LVP (>5 L) [21, 22]. However, there are few RCTs to about, and most of them are small in size (<100 patients). Treatment alternatives such as synthetic colloids and vasoconstrictors have been widely investigated. In a recent meta-analysis on albumin infusion in patients undergoing LVP, 17 trials (1,225 patients, overall) including PPCD, hyponatremia, and mortality as primary end points were identified [23]. Albumin significantly reduced the incidence of PPCD, hyponatremia, and mortality as compared with alternative treatments. Incidence of AKI was reported in 10 of the 17 trials, and a 17 % reduction in the risk of renal impairment was found, though not statistically significant. Since patients with hyponatremia (which develops because of an impaired renal capacity to eliminate solute-free water) show greater susceptibility to the development of refractory ascites, lower responsiveness to diuretics, and higher requirement for LVP, the reduced occurrence of hyponatremia in patients receiving albumin is of potential clinical importance.

16.3 Pharmacologic Properties

The most well-established physiological role of albumin is the maintenance of colloid osmotic pressure (COP). Albumin contributes up to 80 % of the normal COP, due to its high plasma concentration (55–60 % of plasma protein content) and its net negative charge that promotes the retention of positively charged solutes within the intravascular compartment [24]. In addition, albumin acts as an effective plasma buffer thanks to its high concentration and to the numerous charged residues which are present on its surface [24]. Albumin also binds different molecules (including fatty acids, ions, thyroxine, bilirubin, and amino acids), functioning as a reservoir and transporter [25]. The binding properties of albumin also affect the delivery, distribution, and metabolism of drugs [24]. Moreover, albumin has antioxidant properties, primarily due to its reduced sulfhydryl groups (–SH), which are effective scavengers of reactive oxygen and nitrogen species generated during oxidative stress [25]. The ability of albumin to bind free copper (Cu^{2+}), which acts as a catalyst in reactions where free radicals are generated, further contributes to its antioxidant activity [24]. Albumin has also antithrombotic and anticoagulant effects, probably due to its ability to bind nitric oxide (NO) to form S-nitrosothiols. In the S-nitrosothiol form, NO is protected from rapid degradation, allowing for prolonged effects on platelet aggregation and vasodilation [24, 25]. Finally, albumin is thought to play a role in the maintenance of vascular integrity [24] and to exert immune-modulatory and anti-inflammatory effects [19].

Maintaining/improving renal perfusion through volume expansion due to its colloid osmotic properties has probably a key role in the nephroprotective action of albumin. However, other mechanisms such as the prevention of oxidative injury and the binding of endogenous toxins or nephrotoxic drugs may contribute to the observed effects on AKI incidence and mortality [4].

16.4 Therapeutic Use

Albumin, alone or associated with vasopressors, is indicated before paracentesis in cirrhotic patients with more than three admissions per year due to ascites reaccumulation, in addition to sodium restriction and diuretic treatment [26].

In most studies included in the abovementioned meta-analysis of albumin infusion in patients undergoing LVP [23], favorable effects on mortality were obtained with the administration of 8 g albumin per liter of ascites fluid removed. However, albumin may also be effective at lower doses, as suggested by a pilot study directly comparing eight with 4 g/L [27]. These findings might help in reducing treatment costs, but need to be confirmed in further studies.

Albumin infusion is recommended for the treatment of hypovolemia in patients with cirrhosis and AKI according to the International Club of Ascites staging of AKI (ICA-AKI) (Table 16.1) [1]. In patients with ICA-AKI stage 1, volume expansion is recommended for clinically suspected hypovolemia. Crystalloids, albumin, or blood (in patients with gastrointestinal bleeding) should be used according to clinical judgment, after potentially nephrotoxic drugs, vasodilators, and diuretics have been reduced or withdrawn. In case of progression of the AKI stage or in patients presenting with ICA-AKI stage 2 and 3, volume expansion with intravenous albumin (at a dose of 1 g/kg of body weight per day for two consecutive days) is recommended in order to treat prerenal AKI and to allow differential diagnosis of AKI (Fig. 16.1). The maximum dose of 100 g albumin per day should not be exceeded [20]. Differential diagnosis of those cases which do not respond to albumin includes HRS, intrinsic AKI, and postrenal AKI.

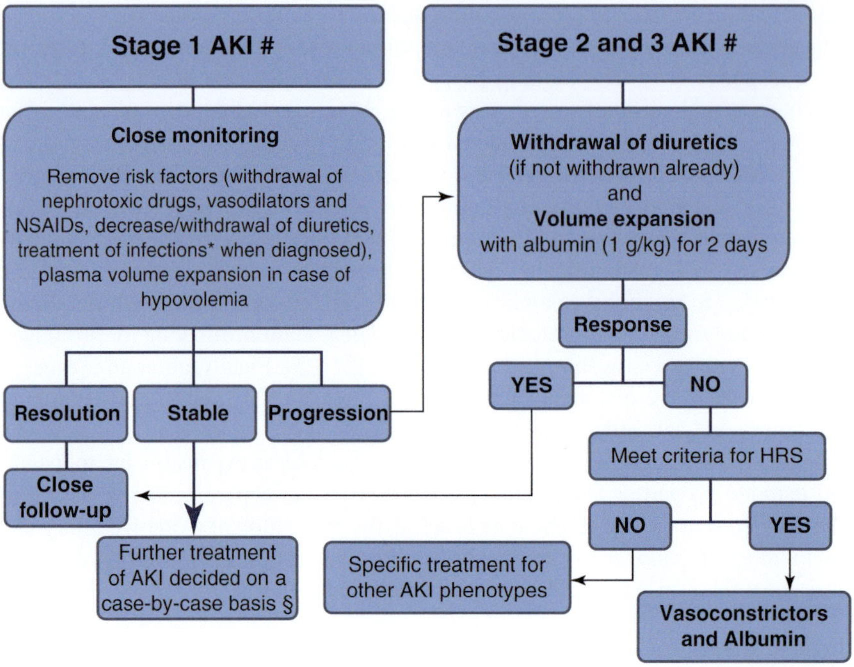

Fig. 16.1 Proposed algorithm for the management of acute kidney injury (*AKI*) according to International Club of Ascites-AKI (*ICA-AKI*) classification that combines "Kidney Disease: Improving Global Outcomes" (*KDIGO*) criteria and conventional criteria in patients with cirrhosis and ascites. *Treatment of spontaneous bacterial peritonitis (*SBP*) should include albumin infusion according to current guidelines. #Initial AKI stage is defined as AKI stage at the time of first fulfillment of the AKI criteria. §No global consensus was reached on this point. *HRS* hepatorenal syndrome, *NSAIDs* nonsteroidal anti-inflammatory drugs, *sCr* serum creatinine (Reproduced with permission from Angeli et al. [1])

Table 16.2 Unconfirmed indications for albumin in liver cirrhosis

Indications	Albumin use
Non-SBP infections	One study available – improvement in renal and circulatory function but no effect on survival
Hepatic encephalopathy	Two studies available – improvement in HE grade observed in one study but not the other
Ascites	Two studies available – better results observed in patients receiving albumin but limitations in both studies prevented a definitive conclusion on the utility of chronic treatment with albumin (answer study currently ongoing)
Acute-on-chronic liver failure	Albumin dialysis (MARS and Prometheus) – beneficial effect on systemic hemodynamics, severe HE, and removal of toxic molecules but no substantial effects on survival

Modified from Bernardi et al. [28]
MARS molecular adsorbent recirculating systems, *Prometheus* fractionated plasma separation and adsorption, *SBP* spontaneous bacterial peritonitis, *HE* hepatic encephalopathy

Clinical Summary

Drug	Indications	Associated treatments	Albumin dose	Cautions	Side effects	Notes
Human albumin solution	1. Large refractory ascites (prevention of post-paracentesis circulatory dysfunction)	Large-volume paracentesis (LVP) with albumin	8 g per L of ascites removed	Albumin is contraindicated in patients with severe anemia or cardiac failure and in patients with a history of allergic reactions to human albumin	Low incidence of anaphylaxis (which may be severe) and hypersensitivity reactions (including urticarial, skin rash, pruritus, edema, erythema, hypotension, and bronchospasm)	To be carried out for LVP (>5 L of ascites)
	2. Spontaneous bacterial peritonitis (prevention of acute kidney injury/ hepatorenal syndrome; mortality reduction)	Albumin in association with antibiotics	1.5 g/kg body weight on day 1 and then 1 g/kg on day 3	As above	As above	According to available evidence, a strong recommendation can be made for albumin administration in order to prevent AKI and to reduce mortality in cirrhotic patients with SBP
	3. Hepatorenal syndrome	Albumin in combination with terlipressin	Not specifically indicated. Previously reported dosages in refs [30, 31]	As above. Terlipressin is contraindicated in patients with ischemic cardiovascular diseases	As above	HRS should be diagnosed by demonstrating a significant increase in sCr and excluding other known causes of renal failure

Conclusion

The most well-established indications for albumin in cirrhosis are prevention of PPCD during LVP in the treatment of refractory ascites, prevention of HRS in patients with SBP, and HRS treatment [28]. According to the literature evidences discussed earlier, a strong recommendation can be made for albumin administration in order to prevent AKI and to reduce mortality in cirrhotic patients with SBP [1, 29]. Albumin may also have beneficial effects on a number of other complications in cirrhosis (Table 16.2), although further studies are needed before any definitive conclusion can be drawn.

References

1. Angeli P, Gines P, Wong et al (2015) Diagnosis and management of acute kidney injury in patients with cirrhosis: revised consensus recommendations of the International Club of Ascites. Gut 64:531–537
2. Egerod Israelsen M, Gluud LL, Krag A (2015) Acute kidney injury and hepatorenal syndrome in cirrhosis. J Gastroenterol Hepatol 30:236–243
3. Sort P, Navasa M, Arroyo V et al (1999) Effect of intravenous albumin on renal impairment and mortality in patients with cirrhosis and spontaneous bacterial peritonitis. N Engl J Med 341:403–409
4. Wiedermann CJ, Dunzendorfer S, Gaioni LU et al (2010) Hyperoncotic colloids and acute kidney injury: a meta-analysis of randomized trials. Crit Care 14:R191
5. Ulusoy S, Ari D, Ozkan G et al (2015) The frequency and outcome of acute kidney injury in a tertiary hospital: which factors affect mortality? Artif Organs 39:597–606
6. Moon KW, Kim J, Kim JH et al (2011) Risk factors for acute kidney injury by non-steroidal anti-inflammatory drugs in patients with hyperuricaemia. Rheumatology (Oxford) 50:2278–2282
7. Downes KJ, Patil NR, Rao MB et al (2015) Risk factors for acute kidney injury during aminoglycoside therapy in patients with cystic fibrosis. Pediatr Nephrol 30:1879–1888
8. Murat SN, Kurtul A, Yarlioglues M (2015) Impact of serum albumin levels on contrast-induced acute kidney injury in patients with acute coronary syndromes treated with percutaneous coronary intervention. Angiology 66:732–737
9. Lee EH, Baek SH, Chin JH et al (2012) Preoperative hypoalbuminemia is a major risk factor for acute kidney injury following off-pump coronary artery bypass surgery. Intensive Care Med 38:1478–1486
10. Kim WH, Park MH, Kim HJ et al (2015) Potentially modifiable risk factors for acute kidney injury after surgery on the thoracic aorta: a propensity score matched case-control study. Medicine (Baltimore) 94:e273
11. Moguel-González B, Wasung-de-Lay M, Tella-Vega P et al (2013) Acute kidney injury in cardiac surgery. Rev Invest Clin 65:467–475
12. Lee EH, Kim HR, Baek SH et al (2014) Risk factors of postoperative acute kidney injury in patients undergoing esophageal cancer surgery. J Cardiothorac Vasc Anesth 28:936–942
13. De Oliveira FS, Freitas FG, Ferreira EM et al (2015) Positive fluid balance as a prognostic factor for mortality and acute kidney injury in severe sepsis and septic shock. J Crit Care 30:97–101
14. Acheampong A, Vincent JL (2015) A positive fluid balance is an independent prognostic factor in patients with sepsis. Crit Care 19:251

15. Wiedermann CJ, Joannidis M (2015) Nephroprotective potential of human albumin infusion: a narrative review. Gastroenterol Res Pract 2015:91283916
16. Finfer S, Bellomo R, Boyce N et al (2004) A comparison of albumin and saline for fluid resuscitation in the intensive care unit. N Engl J Med 350:2247–2256
17. Romanelli RG, La Villa G, Barletta G et al (2006) Long-term albumin infusion improves survival in patients with cirrhosis and ascites: an unblinded randomized trial. World J Gastroenterol 12:1403–1407
18. Bari K, Miñano C, Shea M et al (2012) The combination of octreotide and midodrine is not superior to albumin in preventing recurrence of ascites after large-volume paracentesis. Clin Gastroenterol Hepatol 10:1169–1175
19. Garcia-Martinez R, Caraceni P, Bernardi M et al (2013) Albumin: pathophysiologic basis of its role in the treatment of cirrhosis and its complications. Hepatology 58:1836–1846
20. Ginès P, Titó L, Arroyo V et al (1988) Randomized comparative study of therapeutic paracentesis with and without intravenous albumin in cirrhosis. Gastroenterology 94:1493–1502
21. European Association for the Study of the Liver (2010) EASL clinical practice guidelines on the management of ascites, spontaneous bacterial peritonitis, and hepatorenal syndrome in cirrhosis. J Hepatol 53:397–417
22. Runyon BA, AASLD Practice Guidelines Committee (2009) Management of adult patients with ascites due to cirrhosis: an update. Hepatology 49:2087–2107
23. Bernardi M, Caraceni P, Navickis R et al (2012) Albumin infusion in patients undergoing large-volume paracentesis: a meta-analysis of randomized trials. Hepatology 55:1172–1181
24. Nicholson JP, Wolmarans MR, Park GR (2000) The role of albumin in critical illness. Br J Anaesth 85:599–610
25. Evans TW (2000) Review article: albumin as a drug—biological effects of albumin unrelated to oncotic pressure. Aliment Pharmacol Ther 16(Suppl 5):6–11
26. Lenz K, Buder R, Kapun L et al (2015) Treatment and management of ascites and hepatorenal syndrome: an update. Ther Adv Gastroenterol 8:83–100
27. Alessandria C, Elia C, Mezzabotta L et al (2011) Prevention of paracentesis-induced circulatory dysfunction in cirrhosis: standard vs half albumin doses. A prospective, randomized, unblinded pilot study. Dig Liver Dis 43:881–886
28. Bernardi M, Ricci CS, Zaccherini G (2014) Role of human albumin in the management of complications of liver cirrhosis. J Clin Exp Hepatol 4:302–311
29. Landoni G, Bove T, Székely A et al (2013) Reducing mortality in acute kidney injury patients: systematic review and international web-based survey. J Cardiothorac Vasc Anesth 27(6):1384–1398
30. Martín-Llahí M, Pepin MN, Guevara M et al (2008) Terlipressin and albumin vs albumin in patients with cirrhosis and hepatorenal syndrome: a randomized study. Gastroenterology 134:1352–1359
31. Sanyal AJ, Boyer T, Garcia-Tsao G et al (2008) A randomized, prospective, double-blind, placebo-controlled trial of terlipressin for type 1 hepatorenal syndrome. Gastroenterology 134:1360–1368

Extracorporeal Removal of Serum-Free Light Chains in Patients with Multiple Myeloma-Associated Acute Kidney Injury

17

Gianluca Paternoster, Paolo Fabbrini, and Imma Attolico

17.1 General Principles

Multiple myeloma (MM) is a clonal B-cell cancer of proliferating plasma cells. It represents nearly a tenth of all hematologic malignancies [1]. Renal dysfunction is among the most common complications in patients with active MM, together with hypercalcemia, osteolytic lesions, and anemia [2]. Kidney injury in plasma cells dyscrasias may be extremely heterogeneous. However, only cast nephropathy should be regarded as a myeloma-defining event since all other histological forms should be regarded as different entities related to a monoclonal serum-free light chain (sFLC) production [3].

Renal dysfunction is present in 25–50 % of newly diagnosed MM patients, about 9 % of which needs hemodialysis (HD) [4]. Half of patients with MM may develop renal injury during the course of the disease. Kidney dysfunction can be reversed in approximately 50 % of patients, but the remaining patients will have some degree of persistent chronic kidney disease (CKD). Patients with acute kidney injury (AKI) have higher early and overall mortality. Evidence is accumulating suggesting that

G. Paternoster, MD, PhD (✉)
Department of Cardiovascular Anesthesia and ICU, San Carlo Hospital,
Via Degli Ulivi, 10 Rionero in Vulture, Potenza, Italy
e-mail: paternostergianluca@gmail.com

P. Fabbrini, MD
Department of Nephrology, San Gerardo Hospital, Monza, Italy

University of Milan Bicocca, Milan, Italy
e-mail: paolo.fabbrini@gmail.com

I. Attolico, MD
Department of Hematology and Stem Cells Transplantation, San Carlo Hospital,
Potenza, Italy
e-mail: imma.attolico@tin.it

© Springer International Publishing Switzerland 2016

G. Landoni et al. (eds.), *Reducing Mortality in Acute Kidney Injury*,
DOI 10.1007/978-3-319-33429-5_17

kidney function is tightly related to myeloma cell mass: accordingly, CKD is more common in patients with a large tumor burden [5].

Since the recovery of renal function is associated with a dramatic improvement in survival, MM with severe renal dysfunction at presentation deserves a prompt and aggressive treatment, with the following key objectives [6]:

- Removal or prevention of those factors possibly aggravating renal injury. Maximizing urine output in not anuric patients by optimizing intravascular volume, avoiding loop diuretics, correcting acidosis and hypercalcemia [7], and avoiding intravenous radiological contrast media or other nephrotoxic drugs.
- Reduced exposure of the kidneys to sFLC. Effective chemotherapy is the cornerstone of treatment in patients with myeloma-related AKI. Hematologic response usually translates into renal improvement. Bortezomib, an ubiquitin-proteasome inhibitor, may counteract the harmful effects of FLCs on the kidney through a rapid reduction of sFLC (due to the reduction of myeloma cells) and a reduction of kidney inflammation due to the blockade of NF-κB activation. Bortezomib does not need dose adjustment in patients with renal failure. The International Myeloma Working Group (IMWG) [8] recommended the use of bortezomib-based regimens, including high-dose dexamethasone, as first choice. The combination of bortezomib with melphalan and prednisone may be used in elderly patients with renal disease. In patients with mild-to-moderate renal impairment, lenalidomide may be used as an alternative, adjusting the dose according to renal function. Several studies reported reversal of myeloma-associated renal injury, also in a 20–30% of patients on dialysis who become dialysis independent following treatment [6].

Removal of sFLC with extracorporeal techniques such as plasma exchange has been also described as an adjunctive treatment to further reduce kidney exposure to sFLC and, possibly, to improve renal outcome in patients with MM. However, as discussed below, the impact of extracorporeal sFLC removal (with any technique) on survival is unclear.

17.2 Main Evidence

There is only a small single-center randomized controlled trial (RCT) reporting a reduction in mortality with plasma exchange in patients with MM-associated AKI [9]. Zucchelli et al. [10] randomized 29 patients to receive either peritoneal dialysis or plasma exchange in addition to hemodialysis (HD) and found a significantly reduced 1-year mortality in the plasma exchange/HD group. However, this study is rather old and therapy of MM has profoundly changed since its publication. Moreover, the combination of plasma exchange with HD and the comparison with a different dialysis technique (peritoneal dialysis) make it difficult to attribute the observed benefits to plasma exchange per se [9]. Indeed, more recent studies of plasma exchange in patients with MM-associated renal impairment failed to show any difference in renal outcomes or survival [11, 12].

Nevertheless, new evidence is now available regarding the role of extracorporeal sFLC removal combined with chemotherapy in patients with MM-associated kidney injury [13, 14]. In summary, extracorporeal removal of sFLC is considered reasonable in current clinical practice if it is reserved to patients with cast nephropathy [13] and if it aims to a great reduction of sFLC (60 %) in a very short time (12–21 days from the beginning of treatment) [14, 15].

17.3 Pathophysiological Principles and Clinical Practice

Cast nephropathy is determined by an overflow of filtered sFLC in the proximal tubule that largely overwhelms its endocytic capacity. The high amount of exceeding FLC in the tubular fluid leads to their accumulation within the proximal tubular cells and to intraluminal cast formation into distal tubules [13]. As mentioned, this state is usually induced by concomitant conditions such as hypovolemia, electrolyte/acid-base disturbances, and nephrotoxic drugs, which can impair tubular function.

Therefore, treatment should aim at preventing or removing such precipitant factors, at reducing sFLC production (with anti-myeloma drugs), and, reasonably, at removing sFLC through extracorporeal techniques.

17.3.1 Extracorporeal sFLC Removal

Since sFLC molecular weight is 25 and 50 kDa for κ and λ chains, respectively, even high/superflux dialyzers can barely remove these molecules [14]. Therefore, extracorporeal clearance of sFLC can only be achieved through dialyzers with either higher cutoff (high cutoff and/or plasma exchange dialyzers) or specific adsorption properties.

Plasma exchange has been for a long time the only extracorporeal technique used in cast nephropathy to achieve an effective removal of sFLC through a complete plasma substitution. Three RCTs [10, 11, 16] were performed, two of which [11, 16] found no benefit of plasma exchange on overall survival. It should be underlined that all these studies suffer from several methodological limitations: plasma exchange efficacy was not measured since sFLC assays were not available, patients included had a very wide range of renal failure, and the cause of renal failure was not clearly determined. Furthermore, novel chemotherapeutic agents which have proven effective in the treatment of MM were not used at the time of these studies, and this makes impossible to translate their results into the modern clinical practice.

However, plasma exchange has some conceptual disadvantages. The treatment is short and its efficacy is limited to the intravascular compartment, which may contain only 15–20 % of the total sFLC, due to their high volume of distribution. Moreover, AKI patients often need renal function replacement which is not provided by plasma exchange.

In recent years, other extracorporeal techniques showed their efficacy in sFLC removal [15, 17, 18]. In particular, the new generation of high cutoff dialyzers can provide effective removal of sFLC by either diffusion or convection. Different treatment schedules have been proposed, mainly consisting of daily long dialysis sessions in order to remove as much sFLC as possible. Two RCTs, the EuLITE trial in the UK and Germany [19] and the MYRE trial in France (NCT01208818), are now trying to determine the actual role of these devices, but no results are currently available. All other techniques are anecdotally reported in small case series and, to our knowledge, no RCTs are currently ongoing.

Finally, a new type of high cutoff membrane has been introduced in clinical practice. The Ultraflux EMiC2 dialysis filter (Fresenius, Bad Homburg v.d.H., Germany) was developed to increase the clearance of middle-sized molecules such as cytokines. The filter has a molecular weight cutoff of about 40 kDa (only 5 kDa less than ordinary high cutoff membranes) and allows a lower loss of larger molecules such as albumin or coagulation factors. These characteristics may be of great clinical interest since intensive dialysis with rapid reduction of sFLC but without loss of albumin should be considered as the best goal of extracorporeal therapy. No data have been published so far on this topic. However, our preliminary observations in few patients are encouraging.

Conclusion

Plasma exchange is now not recommended for sFLC removal in patients with MM-associated AKI. However, new extracorporeal therapies, especially high cutoff dialysis, should now be considered for a more rapid reduction of sFLC levels in combination with bortezomib-based therapies. RCTs are needed in order to better clarify the indications and the impact on relevant outcomes of such new techniques for sFLC removal. Meanwhile, we

Clinical Summary

Strategy	Indications	Main evidence	Notes
Extracorporeal removal of serum-free light chains (sFLC)	Multiple myeloma (MM)-associated AKI	The only evidence of a survival benefit comes from an old, small RCT in which plasma exchange in addition to hemodialysis was compared with peritoneal dialysis Other studies of plasma exchange in this clinical setting were inconclusive	Plasma exchange is now not recommended in patients with MM-associated AKI Therapy of MM has profoundly changed in the last decades. Newer extracorporeal techniques for sFLC removal (especially high cutoff dialysis) seem to be promising in addition to modern anti-myeloma drugs (adequate RCTs are needed)

recommend a careful patient selection since only dialysis-dependent patients with cast nephropathy seem to be really eligible to extracorporeal removal of sFLC, and treatment should be tailored on the basis of sFLC levels and efficacy of chemotherapy.

References

1. Kyle RA, Rajkumar SV (2004) Multiple myeloma. N Engl J Med 351(18):1860–1921
2. Knudsen LM, Hippe E, Hjorth M et al (1994) Renal function in newly diagnosed multiple myeloma—a demographic study of 1353 patients. The Nordic Myeloma Study Group. Eur Haematol 53(4):207–212
3. Rajkumar SV, Dimopoulos MA, Palumbo A et al (2014) International Myeloma Working Group updated criteria for diagnosis of multiple myeloma. Lancet Oncol 15(12):e538–e548
4. Kyle RA, Gertz MA, Witzig TE et al (2003) Review of 1027 patients with newly diagnosed multiple myeloma. Mayo Clin Proc 78(1):21–33
5. Blade J, Fernandez-Llama P, Bosch F et al (1998) Renal failure in multiple myeloma: presenting features and predictors of outcome in 94 patients from a single institution. Arch Intern Med 158(17):1889–1893
6. Davenport A, Merlini G (2012) Myeloma kidney: advances in molecular mechanisms of acute kidney injury open novel therapeutic opportunities. Nephrol Dial Transplant 27(10):3713–3718
7. Mhaskar R, Redzepovic J, Wheatley K et al (2010) Bisphosphonates in multiple myeloma. Cochrane Database Syst Rev (5):CD003188
8. Dimopoulos MA, Terpos E, Chanan-Khan A et al (2010) Renal impairment in patients with multiple myeloma: a consensus statement on behalf of the International Myeloma Working Group. J Clin Oncol 28:4976–4984
9. Landoni G, Bove T, Székely A et al (2013) Reducing mortality in acute kidney injury patients: systematic review and international web-based survey. J Cardiothorac Vasc Anesth 27(6):1384–1398
10. Zucchelli P, Pasquali S, Cagnoli L, Ferrari G (1988) Controlled plasma exchange trial in acute renal failure due to multiple myeloma. Kidney Int 33:1175–1180
11. Clark WF, Stewart AK, Rock GA et al (2005) Plasma exchange when myeloma presents as acute renal failure: a randomized, controlled trial. Ann Intern Med 143(11):777–784
12. Gupta D, Bachegowda L, Phadke G et al (2010) Role of plasmapheresis in the management of myeloma kidney: a systematic review. Hemodial Int 14:355–363
13. Leung N, Gertz MA, Zeldenrust SR et al (2008) Improvement of cast nephropathy with plasma exchange depends on the diagnosis and on reduction of serum free light chains. Kidney Int 73(11):1282–1288
14. Hutchison CA, Cockwell P, Reid S et al (2007) Efficient removal of immunoglobulin free light chains by hemodialysis for multiple myeloma: in vitro and in vivo study. J Am Soc Nephrol 18:886–895
15. Hutchison CA, Heyne N, Airia P et al (2012) Immunoglobulin free light chain levels and recovery from myeloma kidney on treatment with chemotherapy and high cut-off haemodialysis. Nephrol Dial Transplant 27(10):3823–3828
16. Johnson WJ, Kyle RA, Pineda AA et al (1990) Treatment of renal failure associated with multiple myeloma plasmapheresis, hemodialysis, and chemotherapy. Arch Intern Med 150(4):863–869
17. Fabbrini P, Sirtori S, Casiraghi E et al (2013) Polymethylmethacrylate membrane and serum free light chain removal: enhancing adsorption properties. Blood Purif 35(Suppl 2):52–58

18. Pasquali S, Iannuzzella F, Corradini M et al (2015) A novel option for reducing free light chains in myeloma kidney: supra-hemodiafiltration with endogenous reinfusion (HFR). J Nephrol 28(2):251–254
19. Hutchison CA, Cook M, Heyne N et al (2008) European trial of free light chain removal by extended haemodialysis in cast nephropathy (EuLITE): a randomised control trial. Trials 9:55

Can Intravenous Human Immunoglobulins Reduce Mortality in Patients with (Septic) Acute Kidney Injury?

18

Lisa Mathiasen, Roberta Maj, and Gianluca Paternoster

18.1 General Principles

Sepsis and septic shock are the most common causes of acute kidney injury (AKI) in critically ill patients [1]. Intravenous immunoglobulin (IVIG) therapy has been suggested to be beneficial in sepsis and septic shock by modulating the immune response, neutralizing bacterial toxins, and stimulating leucocytes and serum bactericidal activity [2]. Commercially available intravenous polyclonal immunoglobulin preparations are derived from human B-lymphocytes and contain highly purified immunoglobulins (Ig), mainly IgG and IgM, with intact Fc portion and with the broad spectrum of activities that constitutes the basis of the humoral immune response. Monoclonal preparations are derived from a single cell line and are directed against a single antigen such as endotoxin or cytokines.

18.2 Main Evidence

Most studies of IVIG therapy reporting data on mortality have focused on septic patients. The only study focusing on the use of IVIG in patients with AKI was a single-center randomized clinical trial (RCT) including 40 patients with mostly sepsis-induced AKI [3]. This study found a significant reduction in mortality in the

L. Mathiasen, PhD (✉)
Estor SpA, Via Newton 12, 20016 Pero, Italy
e-mail: lisa.mathiasen@estor.it

R. Maj
Faculty of Medical Sciences, Vita-salute San Raffaele University, Milan, Italy

G. Paternoster, MD, PhD
Division of Cardiac Resuscitation, Cardiovascular Anesthesia and Intensive Care, San Carlo Hospital, Potenza, Italy
e-mail: paternostergianluca@gmail.com

© Springer International Publishing Switzerland 2016

G. Landoni et al. (eds.), *Reducing Mortality in Acute Kidney Injury*,
DOI 10.1007/978-3-319-33429-5_18

IVIG group as compared with the placebo-treated control group (12 vs. 44 %, $p=0.025$). However, this study is a small, old, single-center study, and after its publication no other studies have reported a significant reduction in mortality with the use of IVIG in the setting of AKI or critical illness [4].

A recent meta-analysis identified 43 RCTs comparing monoclonal and polyclonal IVIG with either placebo or no intervention in septic patients [5]. Among these, 25 studies were RCTs of polyclonal IVIG therapy, 17 in adults ($n=1{,}958$) and 8 in neonates ($n=3{,}831$). In adult patients, ten trials on polyclonal IVIG ($n=1{,}430$) and seven trials on IgM-enriched polyclonal IVIG ($n=528$) were identified. Compared with placebo or no intervention, IVIG resulted in significant reduction in mortality in adult patients with sepsis (relative risk [RR] 0.81, 95 % confidence interval [CI] 0.7–0.93 and RR 0.66, 95 % CI 0.51–0.85, respectively). No significant reduction in mortality was found in neonates in five trials using polyclonal IVIG ($n=3{,}667$, RR 1.00, 95 % CI 0.92–1.08) and in three trials using IgM-enriched IVIG ($n=164$, RR 0.57, 95 % CI 0.31–1.04). This meta-analysis included one large multinational RCT in infants with neonatal sepsis ($n=3{,}493$), which found no benefits from IVIG administration [6].

Eight trials studying the effect of monoclonal IVIG showed no cumulative benefit of antiendotoxin, whereas nine trials of anti-cytokines showed a marginal overall reduction in mortality in adult patients with sepsis.

The results of the meta-analysis by Alejandra et al. [5] are consistent with those of two older meta-analyses [7, 8]. Pildal et al. [7] analyzed 20 trials including a total of 1,711 septic patients and showed a reduction in mortality with IVIG therapy (RR 0.77, 95 % CI 0.68–0.88). However, there was no reduction in the risk of mortality (RR 1.02, 95 % CI 0.84–1.24) when only high-quality studies were included in the analysis (763 patients, overall). The meta-analysis by Laupland et al. [8] included 14 RCTs and found a significant reduction in mortality with IVIG administration in adult patients with severe sepsis or septic shock. The overall beneficial effect on mortality appeared to be more pronounced when higher doses of IVIG (>1 g/kg) were used. Again, the survival benefit was lost when only high-quality studies were included.

In contrast to these results, two meta-analyses using less strict criteria for quality evaluation found a significant reduction in patient mortality with IVIG therapy [9, 10].

Most studies on polyclonal IVIG therapy in adults are small and some of them have been criticized for methodological flaws [11]. The only large RCT ($n=624$) in adult patients showed no effect on mortality [12]. All trials identified to have a low risk of bias showed no reduction in mortality with polyclonal IVIG: three of these used standard polyclonal IVIG [12–14] and two used IgM-enriched IVIG [15, 16].

18.3 Possible Rationale for Mortality Reduction in Patients with Sepsis

The mechanisms of action of intravenous polyclonal immunoglobulins are complex and not yet fully elucidated. It has been hypothesized that polyclonal immunoglobulin preparations contain neutralizing and opsonizing antibodies that inactivate bacterial

Clinical Summary

Drug	Indications	Cautions	Side effects	Dose	Notes
Intravenous human immunoglobulins (IVIG)	*Licensed indications include*: Immunothrombocytopenia (ITP), Guillain-Barré syndrome, Kawasaki's disease, and chronic inflammatory demyelinating polyneuropathy *Off-label use includes*: Sepsis, multiple sclerosis, systemic vasculitis, and rheumatoid arthritis	Too high infusion rate may cause immediate adverse events	*Immediate* Headache, fever, nausea, anaphylaxis, and anaphylactoid reactions *Delayed* Renal, hematologic, pulmonary, and neurologic events *Late* Transmission of infectious agents	0.5–3.0 g/kg BW	Serious side effects are rare According to available evidence, IVIG administration with the aim to reduce mortality in patients with AKI cannot be recommended The effects of IVIG administration on mortality in septic patients are controversial

endotoxin and exotoxins, stimulate leukocytes, and increase serum bactericidal activity. Immunoglobulins may also modulate the release of cytokines and thereby either up- or downregulate inflammatory and immune responses [2]. Both the Ig constant fragment (Fc fragment) and the $F(ab')_2$ fragment have been found to have immunomodulating effects by activating complement and innate immune cells [17].

18.4 Therapeutic Use

Immunoglobulins have been used for more than 25 years as replacement therapy in primary immunodeficiency disorders. Since then, their use has been extended to include a number of chronic inflammatory diseases such as multiple sclerosis, rheumatoid arthritis, and sepsis. Doses of approximately 0.5 g per kg body weight (BW) are used in replacement therapies, whereas higher doses (up to 3 g per kg BW) may be used in inflammatory diseases.

Adverse effects of IVIG can be generally categorized as immediate, delayed, or late depending on the time of onset [18, 19]. Immediate adverse events occur during infusion and may be related to the rate of infusion. Headache, fever, and nausea are common, while more serious events such as anaphylaxis and anaphylactoid reactions are less common. Delayed adverse events occur hours, or even days, after infusion and include potential serious events like renal dysfunction as well as pulmonary, hematologic, or neurologic events. Late adverse events are related to the transmission of infectious agents such as hepatitis C virus [19]. However, IVIG is generally considered a reasonably well-tolerated therapy and serious complications are rare.

Conclusion

The results of clinical trials of IVIG therapy are conflicting. There is a high degree of heterogeneity among studies, some trials using IgM-enriched formulas, while others using non-enriched formulas or combinations. Furthermore, patient populations are highly heterogeneous, with diagnoses ranging from systemic inflammatory response syndrome (SIRS) to septic shock. It cannot be excluded that IVIG may be effective in certain subgroups of septic patients. However, larger well-designed RCTs are needed to evaluate the clinical efficacy of IVIG in sepsis. Currently, there is insufficient evidence to recommend IVIG therapy as an adjuvant therapy to reduce mortality in septic patients with AKI.

References

1. Uchino S, Kellum JA, Bellomo R et al (2005) Acute renal failure in critically ill patients: a multinational, multicenter study. JAMA 294(7):813–818
2. Werdan K (2001) Intravenous immunoglobulin for prophylaxis and therapy of sepsis. Curr Opin Crit Care 7(5):354–361
3. Keane WF, Hirata-Dulas CA, Bullock ML et al (1991) Adjunctive therapy with intravenous human immunoglobulin G improves survival of patients with acute renal failure. J Am Soc Nephrol 2(4):841–847

4. Landoni G, Bove T, Székely A et al (2013) Reducing mortality in acute kidney injury patients: systematic review and international web-based survey. J Cardiothorac Vasc Anesth 27(6):1384–1398
5. Alejandria MM, Lansang MA, Dans LF, Mantaring JB 3rd (2013) Intravenous immunoglobulin for treating sepsis, severe sepsis and septic shock. Cochrane Database Syst Rev 9, CD001090
6. INIS Collaborative Group, Brocklehurst P, Farrell B, King A et al (2011) Treatment of neonatal sepsis with intravenous immune globulin. N Engl J Med 365(13):1201–1211
7. Pildal J, Gøtzsche PC (2004) Polyclonal immunoglobulin for treatment of bacterial sepsis: a systematic review. Clin Infect Dis 39(1):38–46
8. Laupland KB, Kirkpatrick AW, Delaney A (2007) Polyclonal intravenous immunoglobulin for the treatment of severe sepsis and septic shock in critically ill adults: a systematic review and meta-analysis. Crit Care Med 35(12):2686–2692
9. Kreymann KG, de Heer G, Nierhaus A, Kluge S (2007) Use of polyclonal immunoglobulins as adjunctive therapy for sepsis or septic shock. Crit Care Med 35(12):2677–2685
10. Turgeon AF, Hutton B, Fergusson DA et al (2007) Meta-analysis: intravenous immunoglobulin in critically ill adult patients with sepsis. Ann Intern Med 146(3):193–203
11. Almansa R, Tamayo E, Andaluz-Ojeda D et al (2015) The original sins of clinical trials with intravenous immunoglobulins in sepsis. Crit Care 19:90
12. Werdan K, Pilz G, Müller-Werdan U et al (2008) Immunoglobulin G treatment of postcardiac surgery patients with score-identified severe systemic inflammatory response syndrome-the ESSICS study. Crit Care Med 36(3):716–723
13. Burns ER, Lee V, Rubinstein A (1991) Treatment of septic thrombocytopenia with immune globulin. J Clin Immunol 11(6):363–368
14. Darenberg J, Ihendyane N, Sjölin J et al (2003) Intravenous immunoglobulin G therapy in streptococcal toxic shock syndrome: a European randomized, double-blind, placebo-controlled trial. Clin Infect Dis 37(3):333–340
15. Hentrich M, Fehnle K, Ostermann H et al (2006) IgMA-enriched immunoglobulin in neutropenic patients with sepsis syndrome and septic shock: a randomized, controlled, multiple-center trial. Crit Care Med 34(5):1319–1325
16. Rodriguez A, Rello J, Neira J et al (2005) Effects of high-dose of intravenous immunoglobulin and antibiotics on survival for severe sepsis undergoing surgery. Shock 23(4):298–304
17. Schwab I, Nimmerjahn F (2013) Intravenous immunoglobulin therapy: how does IgG modulate the immune system? Nat Rev Immunol 13(3):176–189
18. Berger M (2013) Adverse effects of IgG therapy. J Allergy Clin Immunol Pract 1(6):558–566
19. Nydegger UE, Sturzenegger M (1999) Adverse effects of intravenous immunoglobulin therapy. Drug Saf 21(3):171–185

Part III

Interventions That May Increase Mortality

19 Fluid Overload May Increase Mortality in Patients with Acute Kidney Injury

Ken Parhar and Vasileos Zochios

19.1 General Principles

Development of acute kidney injury (AKI) is common in critically ill patients, most often as a result of sepsis or hemodynamic shock. AKI is associated with significant morbidity and mortality, with published mortality rates in the intensive care unit (ICU) population of greater than 50 % [1]. The prevention and appropriate treatment of AKI is thus a major priority in patients admitted to the ICU.

Intravenous fluid administration is a common intervention in ICU patients, and it is used for both the prevention and the treatment of AKI. Fluid administration can increase stroke volume and cardiac output and accordingly can improve renal blood flow (RBF). Moreover, it can increase mean arterial pressure, improving the perfusion gradient between the renal capillaries and Bowman's space. However, the pathogenesis of AKI is multifactorial and not only due to perturbed hemodynamics but also the result of direct cellular injury as well as indirect injury from inflammation and microcirculatory changes [2].

AKI with oliguria as well as fluid resuscitation often results in accumulation of excess total body fluid. This fluid accumulates in all tissues of the body through third spacing into the interstitial space as well as remaining within the vascular space resulting in increased venous pressure. The presence of oliguria is associated with a poor prognosis; however, it remains unclear if this is due to severity of injury or to fluid overload [3]. It is becoming increasingly evident that fluid accumulation is associated with significant risks and with poor patient outcomes.

K. Parhar, MD, MSc (✉)
Department of Critical Care Medicine, University of Calgary, Calgary, AB, Canada
e-mail: ken.parhar@albertahealthservices.ca

V. Zochios, MD
Department of Anesthesia and Critical Care, Papworth Hospital, Cambridge, UK
e-mail: vasileioszochios@doctors.org.uk

© Springer International Publishing Switzerland 2016

G. Landoni et al. (eds.), *Reducing Mortality in Acute Kidney Injury*,
DOI 10.1007/978-3-319-33429-5_19

19.2 Main Evidence

Several studies have found an association between volume overload and outcome in patients with AKI. A secondary analysis of the SOAP (Sepsis Occurrence in Acutely Ill Patients) study, a multicenter prospective observational trial examining the incidence of septic patients in the ICU, demonstrated that patients with acute renal failure (ARF) had increased mortality and that the presence of a higher mean fluid balance was an independent predictor of 60-day mortality (hazard ratio [HR] 1.21, 95 % confidence interval [CI] 1.13–1.28, $p<0.001$) [4]. Similarly, the PICARD (Program to Improve Care in Acute Renal Disease) study, an observational study of 618 patients admitted to ICU with ARF, demonstrated an independent association between fluid overload and increased mortality which was not dependent on the use of renal replacement therapy (RRT) [5]. In fact, an increased risk of death was shown in both nondialyzed patients with fluid overload at AKI diagnosis (odds ratio [OR] 3.14, 95 % CI 1.18–8.33) and dialyzed patients with fluid overload at dialysis initiation (OR 2.07, 95 % CI 1.27–3.37). This study included a wider diversity of patient conditions (including both septic and non-septic patients) in contrast to the study by Payen et al. [4, 5]. In a prospectively enrolled cohort of 81 patients with AKI requiring continuous renal replacement therapy (CRRT), Fülöp et al. [6] demonstrated not only an association between fluid accumulation and mortality but also a dose-dependent effect of increasing mortality with increased fluid balance. Patients with a volume-related weight gain (VRWG) ≥10 % or a VRWG ≥20 % had a higher risk of mortality as compared with those with a VRWG <10 % (OR 2.62, 95 % CI 1.07–6.44, $p=0.046$ and OR 5.1, 95 % CI 1.22–21.25, $p=0.025$, respectively).

A secondary analysis of the "Fluid and Catheter Treatment Trial" (FACTT) demonstrated that patients with acute lung injury who developed AKI had a higher mortality (regardless of a conservative or liberal fluid administration strategy) [7]. This study demonstrated some evidence of causality, as greater diuretic use was associated with a protective effect on mortality, potentially due to its effect on fluid balance. In fact, when the diuretic effect was adjusted for fluid balance, the protective affect was attenuated, thus suggesting that the observed survival benefit was promoted by the modulation of fluid balance.

Volume overload may influence the natural history of AKI. A retrospective cohort study of 170 patients who underwent dialysis for ARF demonstrated that a higher degree of fluid overload was associated with a decreased chance of renal recovery at 1 year [8]. In a secondary analysis of the RENAL (Randomized Evaluation of Normal versus Augmented Level of Replacement Therapy) study, a multicenter study involving 1,453 patients with severe AKI requiring CRRT, an association between fluid overload and mortality, was present [9]. In addition to this, patients who achieved a positive mean fluid balance had decreased CRRT-free days. A prospective observational cohort study from Finland examining 296 critically ill patients with AKI requiring RRT had similar findings [10]. Fluid overload at initiation of RRT was independently associated with mortality in a dose-dependent fashion. Despite having a lower mean creatinine at initiation of RRT, non-survivors had higher mean fluid balances at initiation and had a higher mean time to initiation of RRT. This suggests that the degree of AKI may not be as critical to outcome as the degree of volume overload.

Oliguria, in addition to volume resuscitation, can lead to fluid overload. Whether these two factors are related or independently modulate outcome remains unclear as several of the studies demonstrating an association between volume overload and increased mortality did not adjust for urine volume [4, 5]. A secondary analysis of the NEFROINT study, a prospective observational study looking at patients admitted to ICU with AKI, attempted to address this question [11]. In this cohort, the investigators found both oliguria and fluid overload to be independently associated with increased mortality, suggesting that both factors play an important role. Further supporting this, the authors also found that diuretic use improved survival, even after adjustment for fluid balance and urine volume.

Another common limitation of trials conducted to date is that they are unable to accurately estimate the fluid balance from hospital admission, due to incomplete or limited charting. In addition to this, the accuracy of fluid balance measurements is questionable given most studies do not account for insensible losses and wound losses. As a potential solution to this problem, a recent study looked at the use of N-terminal pro B-type natriuretic peptide (NTpro-BNP) in combination with bioimpedance vector analysis (BIVA) for diagnosis of a volume overload state in patients admitted to ICU requiring CRRT [12]. Patients with both abnormal BIVA and elevated NTpro-BNP had a higher mortality than those with normal BIVA and NTpro-BNP. However, this study was limited by a small sample size (89 patients).

Most studies to date have been conducted in the general ICU population. Similar findings have been reproduced in the cardiac surgery population, as early administration of fluid can lead to AKI. In a prospective observational cohort of 100 patients undergoing cardiac surgery, those patients in the quartile receiving the highest volume of fluid suffered the highest degree of AKI [13]. Also this study, as the previously cited one, was limited by the small number of patients included.

19.3 Pathophysiology

There are several mechanisms through which volume administration and overload may lead to AKI or worsen outcomes in AKI patients. Fluid administration results in elevated venous pressures and venous congestion. Increased venous congestion reduces the renal arterial-venous pressure gradient resulting in reduced RBF. In a murine model of renal injury, clamping of the renal vein reduced RBF and caused more renal injury than clamping of the renal artery [14]. Studies in swine demonstrated a similar effect of reduction of both RBF and glomerular filtration rate when the renal venous pressure was raised to 30 mmHg [15].

Fluid overload also results in interstitial edema. This subsequently causes tubular leakage and increased tubular pressure, leading to a reduced ultrafiltration gradient. Elevated tubular pressure has been implicated as an important factor in persistent loss of renal function [16]. Studies of patients who have had fluid administration demonstrate an increase in renal volume when examined by magnetic resonance imaging (MRI) [17].

In addition to renal venous congestion and renal interstitial edema, extrinsic factors can impair the hemodynamics of the kidneys. Intra-abdominal hypertension and development of intra-abdominal compartment syndrome (ACS) are known risks of large volume fluid resuscitation due to third spacing from leaky capillary endothelium in the context of inflammatory conditions, sepsis, or large volume hemorrhage [18]. Indeed, AKI is a common complication of untreated ACS [19, 20], in which kidney injury may occur due to impaired renal perfusion from increased renal venous pressure [21].

19.4 Therapeutic Aspects

Although a weak recommendation can be made to avoid a positive fluid balance in order to reduce mortality in patients with AKI, thus far there is no compelling data that preventing fluid overload may be a way to improve outcomes in patients with AKI [22]. Studies looking at diuretic use have failed to demonstrate a benefit to either recovery of renal function or any other outcome such as mortality [23, 24]. There may be several reasons for this. For example, diuretic use may be associated with transient intravascular volume shifts leading to further AKI. Indeed, evidence (though weak) exists that diuretic use may even increase mortality in AKI patients (see Chap. 21). The modality of RRT may also play a role (see Chap. 4), as a systematic review of studies comparing the use of intermittent hemodialysis (IHD) with CRRT did demonstrate a higher rate of recovery of renal function in patients who were initiated on CRRT [25]. CRRT is more likely to be successful at actually achieving a negative fluid balance due to its continuous delivery and hourly regulation of total fluid balance. Like diuretics, IHD may cause much more profound intravascular fluid shifts. Moreover, it is generally less efficient in volume management due to its shorter runs. Finally, protocolized fluid administration has been studied extensively (see Chap. 10). However, a systematic review and meta-analysis

Clinical Summary

Strategy	Cautions	Clinical implications	Notes
Positive fluid balance	May cause AKI May increase mortality in patients with AKI	Only a weak recommendation can be made to avoid a positive fluid balance in order to reduce mortality in patients with AKI	Among strategies which can be used to avoid fluid overload, diuretics and GDT have not been clearly demonstrated to improve outcomes in patients with AKI, while CRRT may provide a survival advantage as compared to IHD

examining studies actively restricting fluid administration using protocol-based goal directed therapy (GDT) did not demonstrate any reduction in AKI with fluid restriction [26]. Further prospective trials need to be conducted to better study these questions.

References

1. Rewa O, Bagshaw SM (2014) Acute kidney injury-epidemiology, outcomes and economics. Nat Rev Nephrol 10(4):193–207
2. Jacobs R, Honore PM, Joannes-Boyau O et al (2011) Septic acute kidney injury: the culprit is inflammatory apoptosis rather than ischemic necrosis. Blood Purif 32(4):262–265
3. Macedo E, Malhotra R, Bouchard J et al (2011) Oliguria is an early predictor of higher mortality in critically ill patients. Kidney Int 80(7):760–767
4. Payen D, de Pont AC, Sakr Y et al (2008) A positive fluid balance is associated with a worse outcome in patients with acute renal failure. Crit Care 12(3):R74
5. Bouchard J, Soroko SB, Chertow GM et al (2009) Fluid accumulation, survival and recovery of kidney function in critically ill patients with acute kidney injury. Kidney Int 76(4):422–427
6. Fülöp T, Pathak MB, Schmidt DW et al (2010) Volume-related weight gain and subsequent mortality in acute renal failure patients treated with continuous renal replacement therapy. ASAIO J 56(4):333–337
7. Grams ME, Estrella MM, Coresh J et al (2011) Fluid balance, diuretic use, and mortality in acute kidney injury. Clin J Am Soc Nephrol 6(5):966–973
8. Heung M, Wolfgram DF, Kommareddi M et al (2012) Fluid overload at initiation of renal replacement therapy is associated with lack of renal recovery in patients with acute kidney injury. Nephrol Dial Transplant 27(3):956–961
9. RENAL Replacement Therapy Study Investigators, Bellomo R, Cass A, Cole L et al (2012) An observational study fluid balance and patient outcomes in the randomized evaluation of normal vs. augmented level of replacement therapy trial. Crit Care Med 40(6):1753–1760
10. Vaara ST, Korhonen AM, Kaukonen KM et al (2012) Fluid overload is associated with an increased risk for 90-day mortality in critically ill patients with renal replacement therapy: data from the prospective FINNAKI study. Crit Care 16(5):R197
11. Teixeira C, Garzotto F, Piccinni P et al (2013) Fluid balance and urine volume are independent predictors of mortality in acute kidney injury. Crit Care 17(1):R14
12. Chen H, Wu B, Gong D et al (2015) Fluid overload at start of continuous renal replacement therapy is associated with poorer clinical condition and outcome: a prospective observational study on the combined use of bioimpedance vector analysis and serum N-terminal pro-B-type natriuretic peptide measurement. Crit Care 19:135
13. Kambhampati G, Ross EA, Alsabbagh MM et al (2012) Perioperative fluid balance and acute kidney injury. Clin Exp Nephrol 16(5):730–738
14. Li X, Liu M, Bedja D et al (2012) Acute renal venous obstruction is more detrimental to the kidney than arterial occlusion: implication for murine models of acute kidney injury. Am J Physiol Renal Physiol 302(5):F519–F525
15. Doty JM, Saggi BH, Sugerman HJ et al (1999) Effect of increased renal venous pressure on renal function. J Trauma 47(6):1000–1003
16. Hellberg PO, Kallskog O, Wolgast M (1990) Nephron function in the early phase of ischemic renal failure. Significance of erythrocyte trapping. Kidney Int 38(3):432–439
17. Chowdhury AH, Cox EF, Francis ST et al (2012) A randomized, controlled, double-blind crossover study on the effects of 2-L infusions of 0.9% saline and plasma-lyte(R) 148 on renal blood flow velocity and renal cortical tissue perfusion in healthy volunteers. Ann Surg 256(1):18–24

18. Holodinsky JK, Roberts DJ, Ball CG et al (2013) Risk factors for intra-abdominal hypertension and abdominal compartment syndrome among adult intensive care unit patients: a systematic review and meta-analysis. Crit Care 17(5):R249
19. Vidal MG, Ruiz Weisser J, Gonzalez F et al (2008) Incidence and clinical effects of intra-abdominal hypertension in critically ill patients. Crit Care Med 36(6):1823–1831
20. Dalfino L, Tullo L, Donadio I et al (2008) Intra-abdominal hypertension and acute renal failure in critically ill patients. Intensive Care Med 34(4):707–713
21. Wauters J, Claus P, Brosens N et al (2009) Pathophysiology of renal hemodynamics and renal cortical microcirculation in a porcine model of elevated intra-abdominal pressure. J Trauma 66(3):713–719
22. Landoni G, Bove T, Székely A et al (2013) Reducing mortality in acute kidney injury patients: systematic review and international web-based survey. J Cardiothorac Vasc Anesth 27(6):1384–1398
23. Karajala V, Mansour W, Kellum JA (2009) Diuretics in acute kidney injury. Minerva Anestesiol 75(5):251–257
24. van der Voort PH, Boerma EC, Koopmans M et al (2009) Furosemide does not improve renal recovery after hemofiltration for acute renal failure in critically ill patients: a double blind randomized controlled trial. Crit Care Med 37(2):533–538
25. Schneider AG, Bellomo R, Bagshaw SM et al (2013) Choice of renal replacement therapy modality and dialysis dependence after acute kidney injury: a systematic review and meta-analysis. Intensive Care Med 39(6):987–997
26. Prowle JR, Chua HR, Bagshaw SM et al (2012) Clinical review: volume of fluid resuscitation and the incidence of acute kidney injury – a systematic review. Crit Care 16(4):230

20 Hydroxyethyl Starch, Acute Kidney Injury, and Mortality

Christian J. Wiedermann

20.1 General Principles

Volume replacement therapy is essential to maintain adequate tissue perfusion and oxygenation in patients with hypovolemia. Crystalloids are inexpensive, readily available, and effective for replenishing both the intra- and extravascular space. However, excessive fluid extravasation with consequent tissue edema is a problem with crystalloid resuscitation, especially in larger volumes. Colloids are more efficient than crystalloids in expanding the intravascular space and can help prevent tissue edema because of better vascular persistence. Compared with crystalloids, the use of colloids is limited by their higher cost and the risk of rare but potentially serious anaphylactoid reactions. Although less expensive than the natural colloid albumin, artificial colloids such as hydroxyethyl starch (HES), gelatin, and dextran display a less favorable safety profile.

HES is a semisynthetic volume expander consisting of carbohydrate polymers of different molecular weights and degrees of hydroxyethyl substitution. HES is marketed as different solutions (with differing compositions) by several manufacturers. Despite a lack of evidence of clinical benefit compared with albumin and crystalloids, HES has been used in a variety of clinical settings to treat hypovolemia including during surgery and after trauma and burns and in critically ill patients in intensive care units (ICUs). Serious side effects of HES due to coagulopathy had already been observed in the 1970s, shortly after it was first licensed. In 2013, medical regulatory authorities limited the use of HES because of safety concerns, including hemorrhage and acute kidney injury (AKI).

C.J. Wiedermann, MD
Department of Internal Medicine, Central Hospital of Bolzano,
Lorenz Böhler Street 5, 39100 Bolzano, Italy
e-mail: christian.wiedermann@asbz.it

© Springer International Publishing Switzerland 2016

G. Landoni et al. (eds.), *Reducing Mortality in Acute Kidney Injury*,
DOI 10.1007/978-3-319-33429-5_20

20.2 Main Evidence

Based on data from clinical studies, HES was shown to be associated with an increased risk of mortality and need for renal replacement therapy (RRT) as compared with crystalloids. A higher risk for other adverse reactions was also reported. These harms of HES were not limited to one manufacturer, molecular weight (MW), or molar substitution and thus probably represent a class effect. In particular, HES-induced AKI was reported in clinical studies independent of differences in product composition. Participants in these trials included kidney donors [1], patients with sepsis [2–4], and critically ill patients [5]. Experimental and clinical studies strongly suggest that toxicity of HES can be attributed to tissue storage: significant doses of HES remain stored in tissues [6, 7], contributing to AKI [1–5] or other organ injuries [8–10], as well as to side effects such as pruritus [11]. Increased risk of bleeding and requirement for blood transfusions due to HES-related coagulopathy have been also documented in ICU patients, patients with sepsis, those undergoing anesthesia for major surgery, and those following blunt trauma [12].

20.2.1 Risk of Mortality

Volume resuscitation with HES has been associated with reduced survival at 90 days in patients with sepsis and septic shock [2, 3]. In the multicenter, randomized, blinded 6S (Scandinavian Starch for Severe Sepsis/Septic Shock) study, 804 patients with severe sepsis (84 % of which in septic shock) were randomized to receive fluid resuscitation with either 6 % HES 130/0.42 (see below), at a dose of up to 33 mL/kg of ideal body weight per day, or Ringer's acetate (RA). 201/398 (51 %) patients in the HES group had died by day 90, as compared with 172/400 (43 %) in the RA group (relative risk [RR] 1.17; 95 % confidence interval [CI] 1.01–1.36; $p=0.03$) [3]. In the VISEP (Efficacy of Volume Substitution and Insulin Therapy in Severe Sepsis) multicenter, two-by-two factorial study, involving 600 patients with severe sepsis, fluid resuscitation with 10 % HES 200/0.5 vs. modified Ringer's lactate (RL), and glycemic control with intensive vs. conventional insulin therapy were investigated [2]. Although survival rates at day 28 did not significantly differ between the HES and the RL group (26.7 % and 24.1 %, respectively; $p=0.48$), the subgroup of patients who received >22 mL/kg bodyweight per day of HES had significantly higher 90-day mortality, as compared with patients who received ≤22 mL kg^{-1} day^{-1} (57.6 % vs. 30.9 %, $p<0.001$). The findings of these two studies were subsequently confirmed in several meta-analyses [13–16] including the increase in mortality in patients who developed AKI after both iso-oncotic and hyper-oncotic HES preparations [2, 17, 18].

The open-label Colloids Versus Crystalloids for the Resuscitation of the Critically Ill (CRISTAL) trial [19] failed to show any difference in 28-day mortality in patients admitted to the ICU with hypovolemic shock randomized to receive colloids or crystalloids for fluid resuscitation. At day 90, mortality was significantly lower in the colloid group (but not following post hoc multivariate comparisons). However, it should be noted that the 90-day endpoint was not included in the original protocol and was added during the conduct of the study. Furthermore, recruitment of 2,857 sequential ICU patients began in February 2003 and ended only in August 2012. Finally, patients in the colloid arm received three different kinds of colloids, rather than HES alone. Due to this, as well as to the high risk of bias, the results of this study add little to the question of HES-related mortality in volume resuscitation.

20.2.2 Adverse Renal Effects

Different mechanisms might be involved in the adverse renal effects of HES, including an increased uptake of starch into the kidneys [6, 7] inducing osmotic nephrosis, tubular obstruction by hyperviscous urine, and renal inflammation [20].

In the VISEP study [2], patients treated with low doses of HES 200/0.5 ($\leq$2 mL kg^{-1} day^{-1}) had a higher rate of renal failure (30.9 % vs. 21.7 %, $p=0.04$) and were more likely to need RRT (25.9 % vs. 17.3 %, $p=0.03$), as compared with patients treated with RL. It was noted that a number of patients received higher than recommended doses of HES (>22 mL/kg/day). However, the higher risk of RRT was also seen in patients treated with HES at the recommended daily doses.

The primary outcome in the 6S trial [3] was a composite of death or RRT need at day 90. Risk for RRT was significantly higher in patients treated with HES 130/0.42 compared with patients receiving RA (22 % vs. 16 %, $p=0.04$). AKI occurred with equal frequency in the two intervention groups. Although 282 patients already had AKI at randomization, this is unlikely to have affected the results of the study. In fact, at baseline, patients with AKI were evenly randomized to the two treatment groups, and the rate of AKI in patients receiving HES did not differ significantly between patients with and without prior AKI at the time of randomization.

In the Crystalloid versus Hydroxyethyl Starch Trial (CHEST) [5], the largest blinded volume therapy study ever performed, 7,000 ICU patients (surgical, sepsis, and trauma adult patients in a ratio of approximately 4:3:1) received either 6 % HES 130/0.4 or 0.9 % sodium chloride (NaCl) in a 1:1 ratio for all fluid resuscitation until ICU discharge, death, or 90 days after randomization. Fluid resuscitation was defined as bolus of intravenous fluid over and above that required for maintenance or replacement fluids. Patients were excluded if they had received more than 1,000 mL of HES before screening. There was no significant difference in serum creatinine levels and urine output between groups at baseline. RRT was administered to 7 % of patients treated with HES and to 5.8 % of patients treated with NaCl ($p=0.04$), confirming an increased risk of RRT with HES. Although indications for RRT were non-standardized, physicians were unaware of study group assignments, making it unlikely that the observed difference was caused by variations in the thresholds for initiating therapy. AKI was evaluated according to the RIFLE criteria (see Chap. 2), serum creatinine levels and urine output: RIFLE-R and RIFLE-I AKI occurred significantly more often in the NaCl than in the HES group (57.3 % vs. 54.0 %, $p=0.007$ and 38.0 % vs. 34.6 %, $p=0.005$, respectively). However, post hoc results showed that serum creatinine levels were significantly increased in the HES group during the first 7 days ($p=0.004$), suggesting a progressive reduction in creatinine clearance. Furthermore, urine output was significantly lower in the HES group ($p=0.003$).

The Fluids in Resuscitation of Severe Trauma (FIRST) study [21] is a small, blinded trial in which 115 patients with blunt or penetrating trauma, requiring 3 L of resuscitation fluid, were randomized to receive either 6 % HES 130/0.4 or 0.9 % NaCl. There was no difference in RIFLE criteria between groups in the 30 days following randomization. However, less renal injury and a significantly better lactate clearance were observed in the HES group for patients with penetrating trauma, but not for those with blunt trauma.

In another small, double-blind, single-center study (Basel Starch Evaluation in Sepsis, BASES) [22], 241 patients with severe sepsis/septic shock were randomized to 0.9 % NaCl or 6 % HES 130/0.4. Volume resuscitation was performed with alternating infusions of 1,000 mL study fluid and 1,000 mL RL until a total amount of study fluid of 50 mL/kg of bodyweight per day was reached for up to 5 days. Primary endpoints were ICU and hospital length of stay (LOS) and 30-day mortality. Secondary endpoints included the course of serum creatinine levels with calculated and measured glomerular filtration rates and RRT need. Use of HES neither significantly reduced the amount of study fluid used nor increased the incidence of AKI. The primary endpoints were also not significantly different between groups. However, the study is most probably underpowered (it is yet to be published and calculation of sample size is unknown). Accordingly, no conclusions about renal safety of HES can be drawn.

The Crystalloids Morbidity Associated with Severe Sepsis (CRYSTMAS) study [23] is a small, randomized, multicenter, double-blind post-marketing study in patients with severe sepsis that compared 6 % HES ($n=100$) versus 0.9 % NaCl ($n=96$). The primary endpoint was the volume of study drug required over 4 days to achieve hemodynamic stabilization. Safety endpoints included AKI (defined as doubling of serum creatinine levels) or requirement for RRT over the study period. Neither the volume required to achieve hemodynamic stabilization nor the time to hemodynamic stabilization was significantly different in the two groups. AKI was reported in 8 % of patients in the HES group and in 10.4 % of patients in the NaCl group ($p>0.05$). Acute renal failure (doubling of serum creatinine levels or need for RRT) occurred in 24.5 % and 20 % of patients receiving HES and NaCl, respectively ($p=0.454$). Additional data on renal outcomes, not included in the original publication, were presented later by the US regulatory authorities [24]: up to day 90, RRT was required in 21 % of patients in the HES group and in 11.4 % of patients in the NaCl group [25]; duration of RRT was higher in the HES group (9.1 vs. 4.3 days); finally, time to RRT also showed a trend against HES [24]. The study was underpowered for renal safety evaluations but renal side effects were still of sufficient concern that changes were made to the US package inserts for HES solutions. This study illustrates the problem of publication bias in clinical HES studies [26].

20.2.3 Safety Data from Meta-analyses

Large clinical trials with low risk of bias suggest that the use of HES is associated with increased risk of death and AKI in critically ill patients. It is uncertain whether similar adverse effects occur with perioperative administration in surgical patients because the trials conducted to date are small and have a high risk of bias.

A review by Van der Linden et al. [27] including 4,529 patients found no differences in mortality, AKI or RRT need between patients receiving HES (mainly HES 130/0.4), and control groups receiving another colloid, a crystalloid, a blood product, a vasoactive drug, or no other treatment during surgery. The number of patients in the included trials ranged from 20 to 203. In general, conclusions on renal safety or mortality differences between HES and crystalloids could not be drawn owing to small sample sizes, differences in comparators, rather small doses of HES, and very short follow-up periods with lacking data from the entire postoperative period [28].

Gillies et al. [29] analyzed 19 studies (1,567 patients, overall) comparing perioperative 6 % HES with clinically relevant non-starch comparators in surgical patients, showing no differences in mortality. Six studies (445 patients) assessed RRT requirement and also showed no significant differences between the two treatment groups. Finally, the incidence of author-defined AKI was investigated in five studies (401 patients) and again no significant difference was found between arms. The conclusion from this meta-analysis was of a more favorable renal safety profile of 6 % HES in surgical patients. However, the studies included were small and with low event rates.

The meta-analysis by Wilkes and Navickis [30] included 15 randomized trials (4,409 patients, overall) that compared HES to non-HES comparators in surgical ICU patients. Fourteen studies used 6 % HES while one (94 patients) used 10 % HES. The CHEST trial [5] provided 65.1 % of the patients included in which 6 % HES 130/0.4 was compared to 0.9 % NaCl. 3.8 % of patients in the HES group underwent RRT, as compared to 2.5 % in the control group. HES significantly increased the risk of RRT (pooled RR 1.44, 95 % CI 1.04–2.01). Similar results were shown in a subset of trials comparing 6 % HES 130/0.4 with crystalloids (pooled RR 1.47, 95 % CI 1.02–2.12). The conclusion of this meta-analysis was that HES increased RRT need among surgical patients.

Using author-defined AKI data from studies included in the meta-analysis by Wilkes and Navickis [30], the pooled Mantel-Haenszel risk difference (95 % CI) between perioperative infusion of HES and non-HES comparators was 1.7 % (−0.4–3.6, $p=0.116$). This pooled effect size for AKI clearly differs from that found by Gillies et al. [29], since the two meta-analyses were based on different trials and had different patient numbers. Therefore, an updated meta-analysis was performed including studies with data about author-defined AKI rate analyzed by Gillies et al. [29] and Wilkes and Navickis [30], as well as two additional studies [31, 32] identified using an updated PubMed search with the same criteria used by Gillies et al. The CHEST trial was not included because patients did not receive the study fluid during surgery but postoperatively in the ICU. The results shown in Fig. 20.1 indicate a trend toward increased AKI events in patients receiving HES as compared with those in the non-HES groups (Wiedermann CJ, unpublished).

Regarding ICU patients, recently conducted meta-analyses clearly confirm the increase in both AKI rate and mortality in HES-treated patients. Zarychanski et al.

Study name	Statistics for each study				AKI / Total	
	MH risk difference	Lower limit	Upper limit	p-value	HES	Non-HES
Diel et al. (1982)	0.061	−0.040	0.161	0.237	2 / 33	0 / 27
Ando et al. (2008)	0.000	−0.174	0.174	1.000	0 / 10	0 / 10
Godet et al. (2008)	0.038	−0.167	0.243	0.717	8 / 32	7 / 33
Mukhtar et al. (2009)	0.000	−0.135	0.135	1.000	1 / 20	1 / 20
Ooi et al. (2009)	0.000	−0.042	0.042	1.000	0 / 45	0 / 45
Lee et al. (2011)	0.019	−0.032	0.070	0.468	1 / 53	0 / 52
Hung et al. (2012)	0.000	−0.048	0.048	1.000	0 / 41	0 / 39
Gurbuz et al. (2013)	0.044	−0.052	0.139	0.370	9 / 74	6 / 77
Skhirtladze et al. (2014)	0.000	−0.024	0.024	1.000	0 / 81	0 / 79
Yates et al. (2014)	0.038	−0.003	0.080	0.067	4 / 104	0 / 98
Kancir et al. (2014)	0.000	−0.097	0.097	1.000	0 / 19	0 / 19
Kancir et al. (2015)	0.000	−0.102	0.102	1.000	0 / 18	0 / 18
	0.021	−0.003	0.046	0.083		

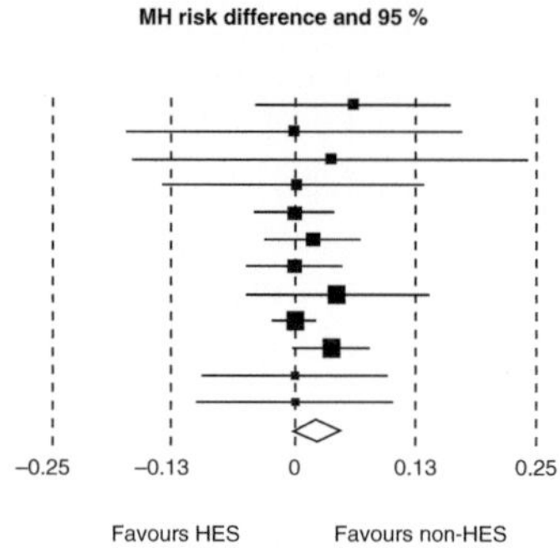

Risk difference (fixed, 95 % CI): 2.1 % (−0.3 %, 4.6 %)
Heterogeneity: χ^2=6.785, df=11 (p=0.816), I^2=0 %
Test for overall effect: Z=1.731 (p=0.083)

Fig. 20.1 Forest plot of author-defined postoperative AKI associated with use of 6 % HES. The meta-analysis by Gillies et al. [29] was updated using the same search criteria in PubMed——"starch[MeSH Terms] OR hetastarch OR voluven OR volulyte OR haes-steril OR hespan OR tetraspan AND surgery OR general surgery"; filters applied were "Randomized Controlled Trial; Publication date from 2013/06/01 to 2015/06/31; Humans"; the reference list of Wilkes and Navickis [30] was also searched. Two randomized controlled trials not included in Gillies et al. [29] and Wilkes and Navickis [30] were identified [31, 32]. The software Comprehensive Meta Analysis Version 2.2.64 was used. *AKI* acute kidney injury, *MH* Mantel-Haenszel, *CI* confidence interval, *HES* hydroxyethyl starch

[13] found that HES was associated with increased risk for renal failure among 8,725 patients (RR 1.27, 95 % CI 1.09–1.47) and for RRT among 9,258 patients (RR 1.32, 95 % CI 1.15–1.50). Haase et al. [33] compared HES 130/0.38–0.45 versus crystalloids or albumin in patients with sepsis. The meta-analysis of nine trials showed a higher risk for RRT (RR 1.36, 95 % CI 1.08–1.72) and AKI (RR 1.18, 95 % CI 0.99–1.40) in patients receiving HES.

20.3 Pharmacologic Properties

Starch molecules are semisynthetic colloids and polydisperse with a wide distribution of molecular weights (MW) [34, 35]. HES solutions for clinical use differ largely in their composition (Table 20.1).

The pharmacokinetics of HES solutions is partly determined by their (mean) MW: the lower the MW, the greater the oncotic effect (and, accordingly, the efficacy in maintaining euvolemia), but the shorter its persistence in the intravascular compartment before glomerular filtration or interstitial absorption. MW of commercially available HES solutions ranges from 130 to 450 kDa. Starch molecules consist of branch polymers of glucose which are made more soluble in water by substitution of some of the hydroxyls with hydroxyethyl residues. This also reduces metabolic degradation by alpha-amylase. HES solutions are commonly classified according to their molar substitution (MS), which is the average number of hydroxyethyl residues per glucose unit. HES is available as tetrastarch, pentastarch, hexastarch, and hetastarch solutions, with molar substitutions of 0.4, 0.5, 0.6, and 0.7, respectively [33].

Table 20.1 Composition and osmolality of widely available solutions for infusion

	Human albumin		Hydroxyethyl starch						Gelatin	
Trade name	Albumex 4[a]	Albumex 20[a]	Hemohes[b]	Hextend[c]	Voluven[d]	Volulyte[d]	Venofundin[b]	Tetraspan[b]	Gelofusine[b]	Haemaccel[e]
Colloid content	4 % Albumin	20 % Albumin	10 % Potato starch	6 % Maize starch	6 % Maize starch	6 % Maize starch	6 % Potato starch	6 % Potato starch	4 % Bovine gelatin	3.5 % Bovine gelatin
MW/substitution			200/0.5	450/0.7	130/0.4	130/0.4	130/0.42	130/0.42	30	30
Sodium (mmol/L)	140	40–100	154	143	154	137	154	140	154	145
Potassium (mmol/L)				3		4		4		5.1
Calcium (mmol/L)				5				2.5		6.25
Magnesium (mmol/L)				0.9		1.5		1		
Chloride (mmol/L)	128	19	154	124	154	110	154	118	120	145
Bicarbonate (mmol/L)										
Lactate (mmol/L)				28						
Acetate (mmol/L)						34		24		
Gluconate (mmol/L)										
Maleate (mmol/L)								5		
Octanoate (mmol/L)	6.4	32								
Theoretical osmolality (mOsm/kg) H_2O	250		308	304	308	286.5	309	297	274	301

Adapted from Mårtensson and Bellomo [34]
[a]CSL Behring (Melbourne, Australia)
[b]B.Braun (Melsungen, Germany)
[c]Hospira (Lake Forest, Illinois, USA)
[d]Fresenius Kabi (Bad Homburg, Germany)
[e]Piramal (Bethlehem, Pennsylvania, USA)

Hydroxyl substitution occurs preferentially at certain positions of the carbon atom skeleton of glucose, with the most frequently hydroxyethylated positions being C2 and C6. The lower the MS and the ratio of hydroxyethylation at C2 and C6 positions, the more susceptible the HES molecule is to degradation by amylase. Since the rate of HES elimination from the circulation depends on metabolism by alpha-amylase, HES molecules with higher MS and C2/C6 ratios are retained for longer within the circulation [35].

After infusion, HES is cleared from plasma by both renal excretion and tissue uptake. Fecal elimination is negligible. HES molecules of less than 45–60 kDa can be filtered through the glomerulus and excreted in the urine. HES can also be taken up by a wide variety of cells and tissues, such as monocytes, macrophages, endothelium, renal epithelial cells, parenchymal liver cells, Schwann cells, and keratinocytes. Intracellular HES becomes incorporated into lysosomes and is resistant to degradation. After tissue storage, HES remains detectable in skin, muscles, and bowel for up to 54, 16, and 14 months, respectively. As a consequence of these properties, the size and number of metabolized HES molecules that remain within the circulation and tissues determine both volume effects and side effects [7].

It was observed that some side effects were more prominent with HES solutions of higher MW, MS, and C2/C6 ratio. Initially, concerns about HES 450/0.7 arose because the possible tissue accumulation after multiple administrations and the prolonged intravascular retention were considered undesirable. HES development therefore aimed at preparations with lower MW, MS, and C2/C6 ratios. It soon became clear, however, that HES 200/0.5 did not achieve the purpose of rapid complete clearance, since measurable HES was shown to persist in the intravascular compartment over 5 weeks after a single 500 mL infusion. In recent years, HES 130/0.4 has been promoted as the new "optimized" standard for HES solutions. Due to its lower MW and MS, HES 130/0.4 might be expected to exhibit shorter intravascular persistence and tissue uptake. On the other hand, its higher C2/C6 ratio (9:1 as compared to 5:1 of HES 200/0.5) would slow its clearance. As a result of these counterbalancing factors, HES 130/0.4 has been found to be equivalent to HES 200/0.5 with respect to volume expansion, hemodynamic effects, fluid requirements, and attained colloid osmotic pressure. Additionally, there appear to be no consistent differences between HES 130/0.4 and HES 200/0.5 in either plasma half-life or maximum intravascular persistence after a single infusion [7, 35].

In a recent meta-analysis of 25 pharmacokinetic studies of HES (including 287 participants, overall) [6], tissue uptake was 42.3 % for low MW HES (≤200 kDa) and 24.6 % for high MW HES ($p<0.001$). Similarly, tissue uptake was greater for lower MS HES (≤0.5) than for higher MS HES (42.4 % vs. 26.6 %, $p<0.001$). Among the three most frequently investigated HES solutions, tissue uptake of HES 130/0.4 (42.6 %) was similar to that of HES 200/0.5 (43.3 %), whereas both showed a significantly higher tissue uptake as compared to HES 450/0.7 (22.2 %, $p=0.001$ and $p<0.001$, respectively). Thus, this meta-analysis did not support the hypothesis that lower MW and MS can reduce tissue uptake of HES.

Tissue uptake of HES is highest in kidneys, where non-inflammatory damage and osmotic nephrosis are held responsible for AKI [36].

Clinical Summary

Drug	Indications	Cautions/contraindications	Side effects	Dose	Notes
Hydroxyethyl starch (HES)	Fluid resuscitation	Critical illness	Acute kidney injury	Lowest possible effective dose up to a maximum of 50 mL/kg. Not to be used for more than 24 h	HES increases mortality and the risk for RRT in ICU patients (especially in those with severe sepsis/septic shock)
		Sepsis	Acute bleeding		Harms cannot be excluded in other clinical settings (no high-quality evidence available)
		Burn injuries	Long-lasting pruritus		
		Renal impairment	Tissue deposition		
		Severe coagulopathy	Severe allergic reactions		
		Severely impaired liver function	Itching		
		Severe heart failure	Increase in serum amylase		
		Hypervolemia			
		Intracranial bleeding			
		Children			

20.4 Therapeutic Use

Strong long-term safety data in surgical or trauma patients are lacking. The fact that no harmful effects have been identified in surgical populations may be the result of poor study quality rather than of the absence of adverse effects in these patients. As stated by the European Medicines Agency, the expected benefits of treatment should be carefully weighed against the uncertainties with regard to long-term safety, and available alternative fluids should be considered [37]. To minimize potential risks, HES solutions should be used at the lowest effective dose for the shortest period of time. Treatment should be guided by continuous hemodynamic monitoring in order to stop the infusion as soon as appropriate hemodynamic targets have been achieved. Finally, patients' kidney function should be monitored after HES administration, and infusion must be discontinued at the first sign of renal injury. Monitoring of kidney function for 3 months after the use of HES has been suggested [37], but this seems impractical, difficult to control, and of questionable impact on patient safety.

HES solutions are now contraindicated in patients with renal impairment or requiring RRT, as well as in severe sepsis/septic shock. HES solutions are also contraindicated in severe coagulopathy and should be discontinued at the first sign of coagulopathy. Blood coagulation parameters should be monitored carefully in case of repeated administration.

The adverse effects of HES appear to be common to all HES classes [13, 38] and to be dose dependent. To date, no safe dose for HES has been defined [34]. In the CHEST trial, an increased need for RRT was observed in ICU patients after an average dose of 5 mL kg^{-1} day^{-1}, one tenth of the maximal daily dose (50 mL/kg) [7].

Conclusion

In 2013, the Medicines Agency and the US Food and Drug Administration determined that the use of HES solutions was associated with an increased risk of mortality and RRT or renal failure. HES is also associated with other serious adverse reactions such as increased bleeding, hepatic organ failure, anaphylactic reactions, and pruritus. For patients with severe sepsis or septic shock, the risks of increased mortality and more frequent use of RRT are considered to outweigh the limited benefits of more rapid attainment of hemodynamic stability as compared with crystalloids. Furthermore, sufficient evidence is not available to indicate that the benefits of using HES in other clinical settings (e.g., during surgery) outweigh the risks.

References

1. Cittanova ML, Leblanc I, Legendre C et al (1996) Effect of hydroxyethylstarch in brain-dead kidney donors on renal function in kidney-transplant recipients. Lancet 348:1620–1622
2. Brunkhorst FM, Engel C, Bloos F et al (2008) Intensive insulin therapy and pentastarch resuscitation in severe sepsis. N Engl J Med 358:125–139
3. Perner A, Haase N, Guttormsen AB et al (2012) Hydroxyethyl starch 130/0.42 versus Ringer's acetate in severe sepsis. N Engl J Med 367:124–134

4. Schortgen F, Lacherade JC, Bruneel F et al (2001) Effects of hydroxyethylstarch and gelatin on renal function in severe sepsis: a multicentre randomised study. Lancet 357:911–916
5. Myburgh JA, Finfer S, Bellomo R (2012) Hydroxyethyl starch or saline for fluid resuscitation in intensive care. N Engl J Med 367:1901–1911
6. Bellmann R, Feistritzer C, Wiedermann CJ (2012) Effect of molecular weight and substitution on tissue uptake of hydroxyethyl starch: a meta-analysis of clinical studies. Clin Pharmacokinet 51:225–236
7. Wiedermann CJ, Joannidis M (2014) Accumulation of hydroxyethyl starch in human and animal tissues: a systematic review. Intensive Care Med 40:160–170
8. Auwerda JJ, Wilson JH, Sonneveld P (2002) Foamy macrophage syndrome due to hydroxyethyl starch replacement: a severe side effect in plasmapheresis. Ann Intern Med 137:1013–1014
9. Schmidt-Hieber M, Loddenkemper C, Schwartz S (2006) Hydrops lysosomalis generalisatus – an underestimated side effect of hydroxyethyl starch therapy? Eur J Haematol 77:83–85
10. Ginz HF, Gottschall V, Schwarzkopf G et al (1998) Excessive tissue storage of colloids in the reticuloendothelial system. Anaesthesist 47:330–334
11. Ständer S, Richter L, Osada N et al (2014) Hydroxyethyl starch-induced pruritus: clinical characteristics and influence of dose, molecular weight and substitution. Acta Derm Venereol 94:282–287
12. Bellomo R, Bion J, Finfer S et al (2014) Open letter to the executive director of the European Medicines Agency concerning the licensing of hydroxyethyl starch solutions for fluid resuscitation. Br J Anaesth 112:595–600
13. Zarychanski R, Abou-Setta AM, Turgeon AF et al (2013) Association of hydroxyethyl starch administration with mortality and acute kidney injury in critically ill patients requiring volume resuscitation: a systematic review and meta-analysis. JAMA 309:678–688
14. Perel P, Roberts I, Ker K (2013) Colloids versus crystalloids for fluid resuscitation in critically ill patients. Cochrane Database Syst Rev CD000567(2):1–73
15. Gattas DJ, Dan A, Myburgh J et al (2013) Fluid resuscitation with 6% hydroxyethyl starch (130/0.4 and 130/0.42) in acutely ill patients: systematic review of effects on mortality and treatment with renal replacement therapy. Intensive Care Med 39:558–568
16. Wiedermann CJ, Joannidis M (2012) Mortality after hydroxyethyl starch 130/0.4 infusion: an updated meta-analysis of randomized trials. Swiss Med Wkly 142:w13656
17. Wiedermann CJ, Dunzendorfer S, Gaioni LU et al (2010) Hyperoncotic colloids and acute kidney injury: a meta-analysis of randomized trials. Crit Care 14:R191
18. Landoni G, Bove T, Székely A et al (2013) Reducing mortality in acute kidney injury patients: systematic review and international web-based survey. J Cardiothorac Vasc Anesth 27:1384–1398
19. Annane D, Siami S, Jaber S et al (2013) Effects of fluid resuscitation with colloids vs crystalloids on mortality in critically ill patients presenting with hypovolemic shock: the CRISTAL randomized trial. JAMA 310:1809–1817
20. Claus RA, Sossdorf M, Hartog C et al (2010) The effects of hydroxyethyl starch on cultured renal epithelial cells. Anesth Analg 110:300–301
21. James MF, Michell WL, Joubert IA et al (2011) Resuscitation with hydroxyethyl starch improves renal function and lactate clearance in penetrating trauma in a randomized controlled study: the FIRST trial (Fluids in Resuscitation of Severe Trauma). Br J Anaesth 107:693–702
22. Siegemund M (2012) Fluid resuscitation is sepsis: is there enough evidence to resolve the controversies? Hydroxyethyl starch vs. normal saline – the BaSES trial. The European Anaesthesiology Congress in Paris, 9–12 June, 01S1, Abstracts, Brussels
23. Guidet B, Martinet O, Boulain T et al (2012) Assessment of hemodynamic efficacy and safety of 6% hydroxyethylstarch 130/0.4 vs. 0.9% NaCl fluid replacement in patients with severe sepsis: the CRYSTMAS study. Crit Care 16:R94
24. Hartog CS, Reinhart K (2012) CRYSTMAS study adds to concerns about renal safety and increased mortality in sepsis patients. Crit Care 16:454

25. Package insert Voluven. http://www.fda.gov/downloads/BiologicsBloodVaccines/BloodBloodProducts/ApprovedProducts/NewDrugApplicationsNDAs/UCM083138.pdf. Accessed 30 May 2016
26. Wiedermann CJ (2014) Reporting bias in trials of volume resuscitation with hydroxyethyl starch. Wien Klin Wochenschr 126:189–194
27. Van der Linden P, James M, Mythen M et al (2013) Safety of modern starches used during surgery. Anesth Analg 116:35–48
28. Takala J, Hartog C, Reinhart K (2013) Safety of modern starches used during surgery: misleading conclusions. Anesth Analg 117:527–528
29. Gillies MA, Habicher M, Jhanji S et al (2014) Incidence of postoperative death and acute kidney injury associated with i.v. 6% hydroxyethyl starch use: systematic review and meta-analysis. Br J Anaesth 112:25–34
30. Wilkes MM, Navickis R (2014) Postoperative renal replacement therapy after hydroxyethyl starch infusion: a meta-analysis of randomised trials. Neth J Crit Care 18:4–9
31. Kancir AS, Pleckaitiene L, Hansen TB et al (2014) Lack of nephrotoxicity by 6% hydroxyethyl starch 130/0.4 during hip arthroplasty: a randomized controlled trial. Anesthesiology 121:948–958
32. Kancir AS, Johansen JK, Ekeloef NP et al (2015) The effect of 6% hydroxyethyl starch 130/0.4 on renal function, arterial blood pressure, and vasoactive hormones during radical prostatectomy: a randomized controlled trial. Anesth Analg 120:608–618
33. Haase N, Perner A, Hennings LI et al (2013) Hydroxyethyl starch 130/0.38–0.45 versus crystalloid or albumin in patients with sepsis: systematic review with meta-analysis and trial sequential analysis. BMJ 346:f839
34. Mårtensson J, Bellomo R (2015) Are all fluids bad for the kidney? Curr Opin Crit Care 21(4):292–301
35. Wiedermann CJ (2004) Hydroxyethyl starch – can the safety problems be ignored? Wien Klin Wochenschr 116:583–594
36. Schick MA, Baar W, Bruno RR et al (2015) Balanced hydroxyethylstarch (HES 130/0.4) impairs kidney function in-vivo without inflammation. PLoS One 10:e0137247
37. European Medicines Agency (2013) Hydroxyethyl-starch solutions (HES) no longer to be used in patients with sepsis or burn injuries or in critically ill patients. 13 Dec 2013. http://www.ema.europa.eu/docs/en_GB/document_library/Referrals_document/Solutions_for_infusion_containing_hydroxyethyl_starch/European_Commission_final_decision/WC500162361.pdf. Accessed 23 Nov 2015.
38. Mutter TC, Ruth CA, Dart AB (2013) Hydroxyethyl starch (HES) versus other effects on kidney function. Cochrane Database Syst Rev 7:CD007594

Loop Diuretics and Mortality in Patients with Acute Kidney Injury

21

Łukasz J. Krzych and Piotr Czempik

21.1 General Principles

Intensive care unit (ICU) patients are often at high risk of fluid retention not only due to underlying conditions such as heart or liver failure but also because they often receive multiple additional intravenous infusions of crystalloids and colloids, including parenteral nutrition, to manage their critical disease [1–3]. Loop diuretics are often used for prevention or treatment of volume overload in patients with or at risk for acute kidney injury (AKI). In addition to the management of fluid imbalance, other acknowledged indications for administration of diuretics in the critically ill include hyperkalemia, hypercalcemia, hyperazotemia, and all their clinical sequelae [1–3].

Since fluid overload is associated with worse clinical outcomes (see Chap. 19), any measure employed to avoid it could potentially improve survival [4, 5]. However, fluid management should be very careful in patients with AKI as overaggressive diuresis may lead to decreased cardiac preload and act adversely on the kidneys. Both hypovolemia (regardless of left ventricle function) and low cardiac output (even with normo- or hypervolemia) result in inadequate renal perfusion, which leads to adrenergic stimulation and activation of the renin-angiotensin system. The resulting vasoconstriction in the renal cortex causes redistribution of renal blood flow in favor of the vulnerable medulla. Hence, the use of diuretics in the setting of AKI should be extremely considerate [6]. Moreover, hemodynamic optimization should be sought whenever possible [7], and fluid management should be guided by the measurement of volume responsiveness using appropriate methods (i.e., central/

Ł.J. Krzych, MD, PhD (✉) • P. Czempik, MD
Department of Cardiac Anesthesia and Intensive Care, Silesian Center for Heart Diseases in Zabrze, Medical University of Silesia in Katowice,
9 M. Curie Skłodowska Street, Zabrze 41-800, Poland
e-mail: l.krzych@wp.pl; piotr.czempik@wp.pl

© Springer International Publishing Switzerland 2016

G. Landoni et al. (eds.), *Reducing Mortality in Acute Kidney Injury*,
DOI 10.1007/978-3-319-33429-5_21

mixed venous oxygen saturation, esophageal Doppler, dynamic parameters from arterial pulse contour analysis).

Loop diuretics may convert an oliguric state into a nonoliguric one [1–3]. This allows the ICU team to apply more sophisticated and complex pharmacological treatments, as urinary excretion of drugs' metabolites is improved. Moreover, urine flow theoretically flushes out debris (including denuded epithelium) and avoids tubular obstruction and backflow of glomerular filtrate into the renal interstitium [1–3]. Altogether, nonoliguric AKI is associated with better prognosis [1–3].

Nevertheless, the protective properties of loop diuretics on the kidneys are unclear, and the use of diuretics in patients with AKI has been even suggested to be associated with an increase in mortality [6].

21.2 Main Evidence

Several observational studies as well as randomized controlled trials (RCTs) investigated the impact of loop diuretics on survival in different settings, including AKI (Table 21.1). Their results were mostly inconclusive and often conflicting. The observational study by Mehta et al. [8] was the only investigation that reported a significant effect of diuretics on mortality. Among 552 critically ill patients with acute renal failure, these authors found an increased risk of nonrecovery of renal function or death in those receiving diuretics (odds ratio [OR] 1.77, 95 % confidence interval [CI], 1.14–2.76).

However, no difference or a nonsignificant trend toward increased mortality was found by subsequent meta-analyses [9–12]. In 2006, Ho et al. [10] analyzed 9 RCTs including a total of 849 patients with or at risk for AKI [10]. The relative risk (RR) of in-hospital mortality associated with the use of furosemide was 1.11 (95 % CI 0.92–1.33, $p=0.28$). It was much higher in patients receiving furosemide for prevention (RR 2.33, 95 % CI 0.75–7.25) than in patients treated for established renal failure (RR 1.09, 95 % CI 0.9–1.31). Also Bagshaw et al. [9] found only a nonsignificant trend toward increased mortality in patients receiving loop diuretics (OR 1.28, 95 % CI 0.89–1.84, $p=0.18$). Sampath et al. [12] summarized 13 studies and found that mortality did not differ between subjects treated with loop diuretics or not (RR 1.10, 95 % CI 0.85–1.42). These results were similar when considering either the eight non-randomized studies (RR 1.09, 95 % CI 0.91–1.25) or the five RCTs (RR 1.12, 95 % CI 0.92–1.35) alone. Finally, in 2010 Ho et al. published an updated review summarizing data on 244 patients at risk for AKI and 632 patients with renal failure [11]. The overall effect on mortality was not significant (RR 1.12, 95 % CI 0.93–1.34), and it slightly differed quantitatively between "prevention" (RR 1.73, 95 % CI 0.62–4.80) and "treatment" group (RR 1.10, 95 %CI 0.92–1.33).

On this basis, the current KDIGO guidelines [13] do not recommend loop diuretics to prevent AKI (class 1B recommendation, i.e., strong recommendation based on moderate-quality evidence), while only a weak recommendation can be made

Table 21.1 Effect of loop diuretics on mortality in non-randomized and randomized trials

Author (year of publication)	Setting	Mortality rate	OR/RR (95 % CI)	*p*	Overall effect on mortality
Non-randomized trials					
Beroniade (1969)	Treatment of RF	LD: 3/12 CTR: 6/12	OR 0.33 (0.06–1.88)	0.21	NONE/NS
Borirakchanyav et al. (1978)	Treatment of RF	LD: 0/6 CTR: 0/8	OR 1.31 (0.02–75.12)	0.9	NONE/NS
Chandra (1975)	Treatment of RF	LD: 5/12 CTR: 3/5	OR 0.48 (0.06–3.99)	0.45	NONE/NS
Mehta (2002)	Treatment of RF	NA	OR 1.68 (1.06–2.64)	NA	INCREASE
Minuth (1976)	Treatment of RF	LD: 47/69 CTR: 12/25	OR 2.31 (0.91–5.89)	0.12	NONE/NS
Uchino (2004)	Treatment of RF	NA	OR 1.22 (0.91–1.6)	NA	NONE/NS
Randomized trials					
Brown (1981)	Treatment of RF	LD: 18/28 CTR: 16/28	RR 1.13 (0.74–1.72) OR 1.35 (0.46–3.96)	0.58	NONE/NS
Canterovich (1973)	Treatment of RF	1st cohort: LD: 15/34 CTR: 7/13	1st cohort: RR= 0.82 (0.44–1.54) OR 0.68 (0.19–2.44)	0.54	NONE/NS
		2nd cohort: LD: 18/39 CTR: 11/19	2nd cohort: RR 0.80 (0.48–1.33) OR 0.62 (0.21–1.89)	0.38	

(continued)

Table 21.1 (continued)

Author (year of publication)	Setting	Mortality rate	OR/RR (95 % CI)	*p*	Overall effect on mortality
Canterovich (2004)	Treatment of AKI	LD: 59/166 CTR: 50/164	RR 1.17 (0.86–1.59) OR 1.26 (0.79–1.99)	0.33	NONE/NS
Grams (2011)	Treatment of AKI (*in ALI*)	NA	OR 0.73 (0.42–1.26)	0.26	NONE/NS
Hager (1996)	Prevention of RF	LD: 6/62 CTR: 3/59	RR 1.90 (0.5–7.26) OR 2.07 (0.49–8.71)	0.35	NONE/NS
Kleinknecht (1976)	Treatment of RF	LD: 13/33 CTR: 12/33	RR 1.08 (0.58–2.01) OR 1.14 (0.42–3.08)	0.8	NONE/NS
Lassnigg (2000)	Prevention of AKI	LD: 4/41 CTR: 1/40	RR 3.90 (0.46–33.42) OR 4.22 (0.45–39.5)	0.21	NONE/NS
Lumlertgul (1989)	Treatment of RF (*in malaria*)	LD: 0/4 CTR: 0/4	RR 1.0 (0.02–41.2) OR 1.0 (0.02–62.3)	1.0	NONE/NS
Mahesh (2008)	Prevention of AKI	LD: 1/21 CTR: 2/21	RR 0.50 (0.05–5.10) OR 0.47 (0.04–5.68)	0.56	NONE/NS
Shilliday (1997)	Treatment of RF	LD: 42/62 CTR: 15/30	RR 1.10 (0.73–1.67) OR 2.10 (0.86–5.12)	0.1	NONE/NS

(continued)

Table 21.1 (continued)

Author (year of publication)	Setting	Mortality rate	OR/RR (95 % CI)	*p*	Overall effect on mortality
Van der Voort (2009)	Treatment of AKI	LD: 13/36 CTR: 11/35	RR 1.15 (0.6–2.21) OR 1.23 (0.46–3.31)	0.68	NONE/NS

AKI acute kidney injury, *ALI* acute lung injury, *CTR* control group, *LD* loop diuretic group, *OR* odds ratio, *RR* relative risk, *CI* confidence interval, *NA* nonapplicable, *NS* not significant, *RF* renal failure

against their use in patients with established AKI (class 2C recommendation, i.e., weak recommendation based on low- or very low-quality evidence) [6, 13].

As mentioned, the renal protective role of loop diuretics is controversial. The meta-analysis by Bagshaw et al. [9] found that in patients treated with diuretics, as compared with control, the mean duration of renal replacement therapy (RRT) and the mean time to spontaneous decline in serum creatinine level were reduced by 1.4 ($p=0.02$) and 2.1 days ($p=0.01$), respectively. Moreover, patients receiving diuretics had a 2.6 times greater chance of increase in urine output ($p=0.004$). Conversely, in their two subsequent meta-analyses, Ho et al. [10, 11] showed that furosemide had no effect on RRT need (RR 0.99, 95 % CI 0.8–1.2 [10] and RR 1.02, 95 % CI 0.9–1.06 [11]). Also the number of dialysis sessions required after pharmacological treatment was not significantly affected by furosemide (weighted mean difference −0,48, 95 % CI −1.45–0.50) [10]. Using a Bayesian statistical approach, Sampath et al. [12] confirmed that the oliguric period of acute renal failure was shortened by the use of loop diuretics (mean difference −7.7 days, 95 % CI −12.5 to −2.08), which was also associated with a high probability of a significant reduction in the number of dialysis sessions. However, there was no between-group difference in terms of time to normalization of creatinine/urea concentrations (mean difference −1.54 days, 95 % CI −5.62 to 2.46).

The use of loop diuretics has been even suggested to cause harm to the kidney and be associated with both renal and extrarenal diseases. In a prospective observational study of critically ill patients, Levi et al. [14] identified the use of furosemide as a significant risk factor for AKI (OR 3.27, 95 % CI 1.57–6.80), also after adjustment for age (OR 1.02, 95 % CI 1.00–1.04) and coexistence of sepsis/septic shock (OR 3.12, 95 % CI 1.36–7.14). In the subset of patients with septic shock, the use of furosemide increased the risk of AKI even further (OR 5.5, 95 % CI 1.16–26.02). Wu et al. [15] found that AKI patients treated with furosemide were more likely to have cardiovascular disease (38.9 vs. 18.4 %), arterial hypertension (42.0 vs. 29.2 %), chronic kidney disease CKD (55.0 vs. 27.0 %), and type 2 diabetes mellitus (17.6 vs. 4.3 %) as compared to subjects not treated with diuretics. Interestingly, only in 27.5 % of cases these conditions were solely associated with the use of diuretics, whereas in 29.8 % of cases a combination of diuretics and other nephrotoxic agents (including antibiotics, contrast media, nonsteroidal anti-inflammatory drugs, angiotensin-converting enzyme inhibitors, angiotensin-receptor blockers, etc.) was present. The degree of renal injury is believed to be positively correlated with the dose of diuretic [9–12, 15], and the risk of AKI is increased by approximately 64 % when diuretics are combined with nonsteroidal anti-inflammatory drugs (RR 1.64, 95 % CI 1.17–2.29) [16]. The great asset of the study by Wu et al. [15] was the opportunity to look into histopathology results of renal biopsies: 58 out of 63 examined cases showed signs of tubular injury or necrosis, out of which 51 showed vacuolar degeneration of tubular epithelial cell and 27 cases showed tubular basement membrane fracture or exposure.

21.3 Pharmacological Properties

The use of loop diuretics to prevent or treat fluid overload is based on their pharmacological properties to increase urine output. Loop diuretics act on the thick ascending limb of the loop of Henle where they inhibit sodium-potassium-chloride (Na-K-2Cl) cotransporter, causing natriuresis. This leads to reduced osmolality of renal medulla and decreased water reabsorption. The inhibition of active sodium transport reduces both oxygen consumption and oxygen metabolic demand of renal tubules. Furosemide also inhibits the enzyme prostaglandin dehydrogenase and causes renal vasodilation with improved renal blood flow. All these effects can theoretically confer protection against ischemic or nephrotoxic injury by improving renal medullary oxygen balance [1–3, 11], although, as mentioned, loop diuretics are thought to possibly cause renal injury [14–16].

Since loop diuretics are largely excreted unchanged in the urine and influence reabsorption from the luminal site, it is the urinary excretion of the drug, not its plasma concentration, that determines the diuretic efficacy. Because loop diuretics are bound to plasma proteins, the reduction in the protein-bound fraction of furosemide due to hypoalbuminemia or the presence of another highly protein-bound drug (e.g., warfarin, phenytoin) increases its volume of distribution, thereby augmenting its external clearance and decreasing urinary excretion. Albuminuria results in urinary drug binding, decreasing furosemide effectiveness [1–3, 11].

Through their renal action, loop diuretics potentially induce hypovolemia, hypokalemia, hypophosphatemia, hypomagnesemia, and metabolic alkalosis. As a weak organic acid, furosemide acidifies urine and reduces the solubility of myoglobin and hemoglobin in patients with rhabdomyolysis and intravascular hemolysis (e.g., due to cardiopulmonary bypass or intra-aortic balloon pump counterpulsation). Aciduria may also promote free radical formation in the urine caused by contrast media. In patients with reduced renal clearance, high-dose furosemide may cause mostly reversible ototoxicity. High-dose furosemide may also induce systemic vasoconstriction. Finally, loop diuretics promote the reduction of mucociliary transport and sputum clearance by inhibiting Na-K-2Cl cotransporter in the respiratory tract [1–3, 11].

There are several drug interactions that need to be taken into account. Loop diuretics reduce the clearance of theophylline, gentamicin, and other organic acids

Clinical Summary

Drug	Indications	Cautions	Side effects	Dose	Notes
Furosemide	Fluid overload Hyperkalemia Hypercalcemia	Preload must be carefully preserved Serum potassium should be closely monitored	Polyuria, hypokalemia, hypophosphatemia, hypomagnesemia, aciduria, metabolic alkalosis, ototoxicity (hearing loss, deafness or tinnitus) with large doses, vertigo, seizures, allergic reactions, agranulocytosis	40–80 mg orally (maximum 600 mg/day) in adults 1–3 mg/kg/day orally in children Continuous/bolus i.v. infusion: initial bolus dose (usually 0.1 mg/kg/h), then adjusted according to the clinical response (usually 0.1–0.5 mg/kg/h)	According to the available evidence, only a weak recommendation can be made to avoid loop diuretics in order to reduce mortality in patients with AKI

(continued)

(continued)

Drug	Indications	Cautions	Side effects	Dose	Notes
Torasemide	Congestive heart failure	Maintain electrolytes during treatment	As above	5 mg (up to 20 mg) i.v./ orally per day maximum single dose 200 mg	The putative mechanism of increased mortality is unclear, but may involve low cardiac output/ hypotension and/or direct renal injury
Bumetanide	Ascites Peripheral edema Pulmonary edema		As above	0.5–2 mg orally once daily 0.5–1 mg once daily (i.v., im) Continuous i.v. infusion: 1 mg/h (up to 12 mg/ day)	
Ethacrynic acid	Ascites Peripheral edema Pulmonary edema 40–80 mg orally (maximum 600 mg/day) in adults		As above	50 mg orally once daily 50 mg i.v. once daily	

(e.g., benzylpenicillin, cephalosporins, oxypurinol, active metabolite of oseltamivir), increase the risk of amphotericin-induced hypokalemia, the antiepileptic effect of valproate, the hypotensive effect of angiotensin-converting enzyme (ACE) inhibitors, and reduce the therapeutic effect of warfarin [11].

21.4 Therapeutic Use

The most popular loop diuretic in clinical use is furosemide (frusemide), and most clinical trials used this drug in the treatment arm [1]. Other loop diuretics available on the market include torasemide (torsemide), bumetanide, and ethacrynic acid.

Furosemide is approved to be used to treat edema in the course of congestive heart failure (CHF), liver cirrhosis, and renal failure and in treatment of arterial hypertension mainly as part of a multidrug regimen [17, 18]. The recommended dose is 40–80 mg per day orally (maximum 600 mg/day) in adults and 1–3 mg kg^{-1} day^{-1} orally in children. The intravenous dose is approximately 0.1 mg kg^{-1} h^{-1}. However, the dose is usually adjusted according to the clinical response. A small dose of furosemide (i.e., <10 mg) can be considered to correct hyperchloremic acidosis induced by a large amount of 0.9 % saline infusion in patients who are not hypovolemic [11]. If intravenous furosemide is used to replace oral furosemide, one half of the oral dose is required. In fact, i.v. furosemide is about twice as potent and rapid than oral furosemide in inducing diuresis [11].

Torasemide is approved to be used to prevent or treat edema in the course of CHF [17, 18]. Its starting dose is 5 mg/day (up to 20 mg/day) given orally or i.v. (maximum single dose 200 mg). Bumetanide and ethacrynic acid are used for ascites, edema, and pulmonary edema [17, 18]. Bumetanide is given once daily at dose of 0.5–2 mg orally or 0.5–1 mg by i.v. or intramuscular injection. Continuous i.v. infusion is usually 1 mg/h (up to 12 mg/day). The dose of ethacrynic acid is 50 mg (orally or i.v.) once daily.

References

1. Bagshaw SM, Bellomo R, Kellum JA (2008) Oliguria, volume overload, and loop diuretics. Crit Care Med 36(4 Suppl):S172–S178
2. Karajala V, Mansour W, Kellum JA (2009) Diuretics in acute kidney injury. Minerva Anestesiol 75(5):251–257
3. Rimmelé T, Karajala V, Murugan R, Kellum JA (2010) Use of loop diuretics in the critically ill. Contrib Nephrol 165:219–225
4. Payen D, de Pont AC, Sakr Y et al (2008) A positive fluid balance is associated with worse outcome in patients with acute renal failure. Crit Care 12(3):R74
5. Bouchard J, Soroko SB, Chertow GM et al (2009) Fluid accumulation, survival, and recovery of kidney function in critically ill patients with acute kidney injury. Kidney Int 76:422–427
6. Landoni G, Bove T, Székely A et al (2013) Reducing mortality in acute kidney injury patients: systematic review and international web-based survey. J Cardiothorac Vasc Anesth 27(6):1384–1398

7. Brienza N, Giglio MT, Marucci M, Fiore T (2009) Does perioperative hemodynamic optimization protect renal function in surgical patients? A meta-analytic study. Crit Care Med 37(6):2079–2090
8. Mehta RL, Pascual MT, Soroko S, Chertow GM, PICARD Study Group (2002) Diuretics, mortality, and nonrecovery of renal function in acute renal failure. JAMA 288(20):2547–2553
9. Bagshaw SM, Delaney A, Haase M et al (2007) Loop diuretics in the management of acute renal failure: a systematic review and meta-analysis. Crit Care Resusc 9:60–68
10. Ho KM, Sheridan DJ (2006) Meta-analysis of frusemide to prevent or treat acute renal failure. BMJ 333:420
11. Ho KM, Power BM (2010) Benefits and risks of furosemide in acute kidney injury. Anaesthesia 65(3):283–293
12. Sampath S, Moran JL, Graham PL et al (2007) The efficacy of loop diuretics in acute renal failure: assessment using Bayesian evidence synthesis techniques. Crit Care Med 35(11):2516–2524
13. Kidney Disease: Improving Global Outcomes (KDIGO) Acute Kidney Injury Work Group (2012) KDIGO clinical practice guideline for acute kidney injury. Kidney Inter Suppl 2:1–138
14. Levi TM, Rocha MS, Almeida DN et al (2012) Furosemide is associated with acute kidney injury in critically ill patients. Braz J Med Biol Res 45(9):827–833
15. Wu X, Zhang W, Ren H et al (2014) Diuretics associated acute kidney injury: clinical and pathological analysis. Ren Fail 36(7):1051–1055
16. Dreischulte T, Morales DR, Bell S, Guthrie B (2015) Combined use of nonsteroidal anti-inflammatory drugs with diuretics and/or renin-angiotensin system inhibitors in the community increases the risk of acute kidney injury. Kidney Int 88(2):396–403
17. Oh SW, Han SY (2015) Loop diuretics in clinical practice. Electrolyte Blood Press 13(1):17–21
18. Roush GC, Kaur R, Ernst ME (2014) Diuretics: a review and update. J Cardiovasc Pharmacol Ther 19(1):5–13

Part IV
Update

Reducing Mortality in Patients with Acute Kidney Injury: A Systematic Update

22

Marta Mucchetti, Federico Masserini, and Luigi Verniero

22.1 Introduction

Acute kidney injury (AKI) is a major concern in critically ill patients. Despite considerable progress, up to 67 % of intensive care unit (ICU) patients develop some degree of AKI, and 5–6 % require renal replacement therapy (RRT). Moreover, AKI and RRT correlate with an increased risk of death [1]. The first international web-based Consensus Conference on mortality reduction in patients with or at risk for AKI (see Chap. 3) [1] specifically addressed this issue and identified the 18 drugs, techniques, and strategies which are discussed in this book.

As described in detail in Chap. 3, this process is made up of three fundamental components: (a) a systematic literature search, (b) the evaluation of the selected papers during an expert meeting, and (c) the validation of the selected interventions through an international web vote. This approach has been named "Democracy-Based Medicine" and is meant to integrate the traditional "Evidence-Based Medicine," especially in those settings such as intensive care where it cannot give strong recommendations, due to the lack of high-quality evidence [2, 3].

Since literature is constantly evolving, systematic updates are needed to confirm or challenge the validity of the selected interventions and to evaluate new ones. In this chapter, we report all papers that have been published since the

M. Mucchetti, MD (✉)
Department of Anesthesia and Intensive Care, San Raffaele Scientific Institute,
Via Olgettina, 60, Milan 20132, Italy
e-mail: marta.mucchetti@gmail.com

F. Masserini
Faculty of Medical Sciences, Vita-Salute San Raffaele University, Milan, Italy

L. Verniero, MD
Cardiac Anesthesia and Intensive Care Unit, A.O.R.N. "Dei Colli" – Monaldi Hospital,
Naples, Italy

© Springer International Publishing Switzerland 2016

G. Landoni et al. (eds.), *Reducing Mortality in Acute Kidney Injury*,
DOI 10.1007/978-3-319-33429-5_22

Consensus Conference was held and that show a significant effect on mortality in patients with AKI.

22.2 Methods

A sensitive PubMed search was performed to systematically identify all papers dealing with interventions influencing survival in patients with AKI, published since February 15, 2012. The same search strategy of the Consensus Conference was used (Box 22.1). The search was updated on July 1, 2015. Further topics were identified by cross-checking of references.

Box 22.1. The Full Search Strategy Used to Identify All Studies Reporting a Significant Effect on Mortality in Patients with AKI

((acute AND (renal OR kidney) AND (failure OR injury)) OR (renal AND replacement AND therapy)) AND ((death* OR survival OR mortality)) AND (prevent* OR reducti* OR reduci*) AND (significat* OR significan*) AND (randomized controlled trial[pt] OR controlled clinical trial[pt] OR randomized controlled trials[mh] OR random allocation[mh] OR double-blind method[mh] OR single-blind method[mh] OR clinical trial[pt] OR clinical trials[mh] OR (clinical trial[tw] OR ((singl*[tw] OR doubl*[tw] OR trebl*[tw] OR tripl*[tw]) AND (mask*[tw] OR blind[tw])) OR (latin square[tw]) OR placebos[mh] OR placebo*[tw] OR random*[tw] OR research design[mh:noexp] OR comparative study[tw] OR follow-up studies[mh] OR prospective studies[mh] OR cross-over studies[mh] OR control*[tw] OR prospectiv*[tw] OR volunteer*[tw]) NOT (animal[mh] NOT human[mh]))

Papers were selected if they fulfilled all the following criteria: (a) published in a peer-reviewed journal, (b) dealt with adult patients with or at risk for AKI, and (c) reported a statistically significant reduction or increase in mortality.

22.3 Intervention That Might Influence Survival in Patients with or at Risk for AKI

The systematic search yielded 224 results. By screening titles and abstracts, 201 papers were excluded, and the remaining 23 were carefully read. Seven further papers were excluded. Finally, 13 studies [4–16], dealing with 10 different interventions, were included in the present update (Table 22.1).

Seven new interventions have been found to possibly improve survival. In cardiac surgery patients, the preoperative administration of renin-angiotensin system inhibitors (RAS-I) [4] and of aspirin [5], the intraoperative use of aprotinin [6], and the use of dexmedetomidine after cardiopulmonary bypass (CPB) [7] showed some

Table 22.1 The 13 studies dealing with interventions with a significant effect on mortality in patients with or at risk for AKI published after the Consensus Conference

Refs.	Author	Type of evidence	Drug/technique/ strategy	Control	Setting
Improve survival					
[4]	Shi (2013)	Retrospective cohort study	Preoperative RAS-I	Nothing	Cardiac surgery
[5]	Yao (2015)	Retrospective cohort study	Aspirin within the 5 days preceding surgery	Nothing	Cardiac surgery
[6]	Walkden (2013)	Retrospective case-control study	Aprotinin on the market	Aprotinin withdrawal from the market	Cardiac surgery
[7]	Ji (2013)	Retrospective cohort study	Sedation with dexmedetomidine after CPB	Other sedatives	Cardiac surgery
[8]	Spini (2013)	Prospective interventional study	CRRT pre- and post-PCI	CRRT post-PCI	Contrast-induced nephropathy after primary PCI in patients with CKD
[9]	Wang (2014)	Post hoc analysis of an mRCT (RENAL study)	ACEI	Nothing	AKI needing renal replacement therapy
[10]	Guo (2014)	Prospective cohort study	Short-term high-volume hemofiltration	Optimal standard therapy	Severe acute pancreatitis
Increase mortality					
[11]	Bellomo (2012)	Post hoc analysis of an mRCT (RENAL study)	Positive mean fluid balance within 28 day	Null or negative balance	Critically ill patients with AKI
[12]	Vaara (2012)	Retrospective cohort study	>10 % of body weight at initiation of dialysis	<10 % of body weight at initiation of dialysis	Critically ill patients in RRT
[13]	Silversides (2014)	Prospective cohort study	>10 % of body weight at initiation of dialysis	<10 % of body weight at initiation of dialysis	Critically ill patients in RRT
[14]	Zhang (2015)	Meta-analysis of retrospective/ cohort studies	Fluid overload	Null or negative balance	Critically ill patients with AKI

(continued)

Table 22.1 (continued)

Refs.	Author	Type of evidence	Drug/technique/ strategy	Control	Setting
[15]	Manari (2014)	mRCT	High-volume hydration	Standard volume hydration	Contrast-induced nephropathy after primary PCI
[16]	Haase (2013)	mRCT	Prophylactic sodium bicarbonate	Sodium chloride	Cardiac surgery

ACEI angiotensin-converting enzyme inhibitor, *AKI* acute kidney injury, *CKD* chronic kidney disease, *CPB* cardiopulmonary bypass, *CRRT* continuous renal replacement therapy, *mRCT* multicenter randomized controlled trial, *PCI* percutaneous coronary intervention, *RAS-I* renin-angiotensin system inhibitor, *RRT* renal replacement therapy

beneficial effect on both renal function and survival. Similarly, the use of continuous renal replacement therapy (CRRT) both before and after percutaneous coronary intervention (PCI) might be more effective in preventing contrast-induced nephropathy (CIN) and improving long-term survival than CRRT performed only after the procedure [8]. The use of angiotensin-converting enzyme inhibitors (ACEI) in patients with AKI needing RRT showed some dubious beneficial effect [9]. Finally, a short-term course of high-volume hemofiltration (HVHF) in severe acute pancreatitis (SAP) may reduce renal complications and mortality [10].

Three interventions were shown (or confirmed) to increase mortality in patients with or at high risk for AKI: positive fluid balance in critically ill patients with AKI [11–14], high-volume hydration to prevent CIN after primary PCI [15], and prophylactic sodium bicarbonate in cardiac surgery [16].

The quality of the selected evidence was low. Only two studies were randomized controlled trials (RCTs) [15, 16], two were post hoc analyses of a large multicenter RCT [9, 11], and the remaining were retrospective [4–7, 12] or prospective [8, 10, 13] cohort or case-control studies and a meta-analysis of cohort studies [14].

Only positive fluid balance [11–14] and RRT to prevent CIN [8] were already selected and discussed by the 2012 Consensus Conference [1].

22.3.1 Interventions That Might Improve Survival

22.3.1.1 Preoperative Renin-Angiotensin System Inhibitors in Cardiac Surgery

RAS-I, including ACEI, angiotensin-receptor blockers, and antialdosterone drugs, can provide end-organ protection in patients with cardiovascular and renal disease. Nevertheless, perioperative studies remain few and inconclusive. Only one study found a survival benefit in this context. Shi et al. [4] performed a retrospective cohort study involving 2,322 patients who underwent on-pump cardiac surgery at a single US medical center over a 10-year period (2001–2011). Patients were divided into two groups, which were compared afterward: one formed by patients treated for at least 2 weeks before surgery with RAS-I (RAS-I group) and the other formed by the remaining patients (non-RAS-I group). The RAS-I group showed a higher incidence of diabetes and cardiovascular diseases/medications. Despite this, operative mortality (defined as in-hospital or 30-day mortality) was lower in the RAS-I group (2.99 %) as compared to the non-RAS-I group (4.62 %) (odds ratio [OR] 0.636, 95 % confidence interval [CI] 0.42–0.981, $p=0.039$). The overall incidence of AKI was also reduced (27.2 % vs. 34 %, OR 0.726, 95 % CI 0.60–0.87, $p=0.0007$), although the difference was statistically significant only for AKI stage I but no for stages II and III (see Chap. 2). In this study, RAS-I also reduced the incidence of septicemia.

22.3.1.2 Preoperative Aspirin in Patients with Chronic Kidney Disease Undergoing Cardiac Surgery

The administration of aspirin before surgery represents a balance between preventing perioperative thrombotic events and promoting surgical bleeding. Few studies suggested that it could improve cardiovascular and renal outcome. In particular, aspirin might protect kidneys from the ischemia/reperfusion injury induced by cardiac surgery. Yao et al. [5] performed a retrospective cohort study on the effect of preoperative aspirin in patients with chronic kidney disease (CKD) undergoing cardiac surgery. They analyzed data from 3,585 patients that were treated in two tertiary medical centers between 2001 and 2010. On the basis of the preoperative (i.e., 5 days before surgery) use of aspirin or not, patients were divided into two groups. The same patient population was also classified in five groups according to baseline kidney function (from normal to dialysis). Patients in the aspirin group had a significant lower risk to develop AKI (OR 0.533, 95 % CI 0.466–0.636, $p<0.001$). The use of aspirin did not show any significant effect on 30-day mortality in patients with normal renal function or mild CKD. Conversely, a survival benefit was detected in patients with moderate, severe, or end-stage kidney disease (i.e., estimated glomerular filtration rate [eGFR] <60 mL/min/1.73 m^2).

However, the only high-quality trial on this subject was performed in noncardiac surgery and did not show any positive effect of aspirin on postoperative renal function or mortality [17]. Moreover, severe bleeding was associated with an increased risk of AKI.

22.3.1.3 Aprotinin in Cardiac Surgery

Aprotinin is a serine protease inhibitor with broad anti-inflammatory and prohemostatic effects. It was initially licensed for high-risk coronary artery bypass graft (CABG) surgery. Between 2005 and 2008, several large observational studies reported an association between aprotinin use and AKI, myocardial infarction, and stroke. These safety concerns led to the drug withdrawal from the market after the publication, in 2008, of the BART trial [18], which found an apparent increase in mortality in the aprotinin group when compared with patients receiving lysine analogues. Aprotinin was reintroduced in Europe and Canada in 2010, although with very strict indications, after the subsequent revisiting of the BART study data raised questions as to the validity of this safety signal.

Walkden et al. [6] analyzed retrospectively the data from 8,795 patients who underwent cardiac surgery at the Bristol Royal Infirmary between 2005 and 2010. Patients were divided into two cohorts according to whether they had undergone surgery before or after aprotinin withdrawal: the first group ($n=3{,}578$) had undergone surgery between January 1, 2005, and June 30, 2007, and the second ($n=3{,}030$) between January 1, 2009, and December 31, 2010. The patients who underwent surgery between July 1, 2007, and December 31, 2008, were not included in the study. Aprotinin withdrawal was associated with an increase in blood losses, transfusion requirements, and re-sternotomy. While postoperative cardiac, pulmonary, and infectious morbidity decreased, the incidence of postoperative AKI increased from 23.4 % to 36.2 % (OR 1.86, 95 % CI 1.53–2.25). A trend toward increased all-cause mortality was evident in the first postoperative month following the withdrawal of the drug. The relative increase in mortality was significant among high-risk patients (hazard ratio [HR] 2.51, 95 % CI 1.00–6.29). Despite the limitations related to the "before and after" nested case-control design, these findings mirror those of other similar studies from Europe, North America, and Asia.

22.3.1.4 Sedation with Dexmedetomidine After On-Pump Cardiac Surgery

Dexmedetomidine is a highly selective short-acting intravenous alpha-2 agonist, used as a sedative drug. Ji et al. [7] hypothesized that it can have a nephroprotective role in cardiac surgery by reducing sympathetic activation, and the consequent hemodynamic instability, after CPB. They conducted a retrospective cohort study involving 1,219 consecutive patients who underwent cardiac surgery at a single tertiary medical center from 2006 to 2011. The 1,133 patients identified were split into two groups: those who received dexmedetomidine and those who did not receive the drug over the post-CPB period. The use of dexmedetomidine after CPB was associated with a reduction in postoperative AKI (adjusted OR 0.70, 95 % CI 0.54–0.92, $p=0.0089$), particularly in patients with normal preoperative kidney function or mild CKD. Dexmedetomidine was also associated with a decrease in postoperative in-hospital and 30-day mortality (adjusted OR 0.34, 95 % CI 0.19–0.61, $p<0.0001$ and adjusted OR 0.39, 95 % CI 0.23–0.66, $p<0.0001$, respectively).

This is the first and so far only study exploring the correlation between dexmedetomidine use and AKI in cardiac surgery.

22.3.1.5 Continuous Renal Replacement Therapy Before and After Percutaneous Coronary Intervention in Patients with Chronic Kidney Disease

CIN is a major cause of morbidity and mortality in patients undergoing PCI, and it is more likely to develop in those with preexisting CKD. In the 2012 Consensus Conference, only two studies were identified in this setting: one on peri-angiography

CRRT (see Chap. 8) and the other on N-acetylcysteine (see Chap. 12). In both cases, the Consensus Conference expressed only a weak recommendation, due to the lack of confirmation of these results in subsequent trials and meta-analyses [1].

In a small retrospective cohort study, Spini et al. [8] enrolled 46 consecutive patients with CKD who underwent PCI. Patients were treated according to two different protocols: the $CRRT_{pre\text{-}post}$ group received CRRT at least 6 h before and 24 h after contrast medium administration, while the $CRRT_{post}$ group was treated only after the procedure. Demographic features of the two groups were similar. The researchers did not observe any significant difference in serum creatinine levels and eGFR at discharge, but during long-term follow-up the $CRRT_{pre\text{-}post}$ group showed a lower percentage of CKD worsening (12 % vs. 43 %, $p=0.042$) and a lower mortality rate (16 % vs. 57 %, $p=0.009$).

A complete overview on this topic can be found in Chap. 8.

22.3.1.6 Angiotensin-Converting Enzyme Inhibitors in Patients with Acute Kidney Injury Needing Renal Replacement Therapy

ACEI are widespread used to slow the progression of CKD, and current guidelines recommend their use in patients on chronic hemodialysis with congestive heart failure. Nevertheless, the use of ACEI in patients with AKI is still controversial, with available literature consisting in few low-quality studies performed in cardiac surgery (see paragraph 22.3.1.1).

Using the data of a large multicenter RCT [18], Wang et al. [9] conducted a prospective observational study which assessed for the first time the association between ACEI and AKI in critically ill patients needing RRT. Complete data on ACEI use were available for 1,463 patients, among whom 9.7 % received ACEI at least once during the study period. Patients treated with ACEI were significantly older ($p=0.02$) and had a lower APACHE III score ($p=0.03$) and sepsis rate ($p<0.001$) at baseline. The use of ACEI was independently associated with decreased 90-day mortality (HR 0.46, 95 % CI 0.30–0.71, $p<0.001$) when adjusted for baseline variables. In addition, ACEI use was associated with lower 28-day mortality (HR 0.38, 95 % CI 0.23–0.63, $p<0.001$) and higher RRT-free days ($p=0.001$). However, statistical significance on mortality was lost when the analysis was adjusted for time-dependent covariates (HR for 90-day mortality 0.78, 95 %CI 0.51–1.21, $p=0.3$). This topic certainly deserves further investigation.

22.3.1.7 Short-Term Continuous High-Volume Hemofiltration in Severe Acute Pancreatitis

The systemic inflammatory response contributes to the severity of SAP. Therefore, different blood purification modalities have been tested in order to reduce morbidity and mortality in these patients, by removing cytokines from circulation.

Guo et al. [10] conducted a prospective cohort study on the prophylactic use of HVHF in patients with SAP and without preexisting AKI. Sixty-one patients were enrolled and alternately allocated in a 1:1 ratio to either 72 h of continuous HVHF or conventional treatment. The authors observed a reduction in both morbidity and mortality. Renal failure (RF) was defined as a serum creatinine >170 μmol/L (2 mg/dL). The incidence of RF (15.6 % vs. 44.8 %, $p<0.013$) and its mean duration (7.9 ± 8.5 days vs. 15.6 ± 12.4, $p<0.001$) were significantly reduced in the HVHF group. Also mortality seemed to be positively affected by this strategy (25 % vs. 51.7 %, $p=0.033$).

22.3.2 Interventions That Might Increase Mortality

22.3.2.1 Positive Fluid Balance in Acute Kidney Injury

On the basis of two observational studies, the Consensus Conference made a weak recommendation to avoid positive fluid balance in patients with AKI [1]. Since then, other three observational studies [11–13] and a meta-analysis [14] confirmed the deleterious effects of fluid overload in critically ill patients with AKI. The main findings of these studies are briefly reported below, while a detailed discussion on this topic can be found in Chap. 19.

Bellomo et al. [11] conducted a secondary analysis of the RENAL study data [19] focusing on the relationship between fluid balance and 90-day mortality. Complete data on fluid balance were available for 1,453 patients, and both daily and cumulative fluid balance was studied. During ICU stay, daily fluid balance among survivors was −234 mL as compared to +560 mL among non-survivors ($p<0.0001$). Mean cumulative fluid balance over the same period was −941 and +1,755 mL, respectively ($p=0.0003$). A negative mean daily fluid balance during study treatment was independently associated with a decreased risk of death at 90 days (OR 0.318, 95 % CI 0.24–0.43, $p<0.000.1$). In addition, a negative mean daily fluid balance was associated with significantly increased RRT-free days ($p=0.0017$).

A correlation between fluid overload and mortality was shown by Vaara et al. [12] and Silversides et al. [13] in two large observational studies. In both investigations, the authors defined fluid overload at RRT initiation as a cumulative weight gain >10 % compared to admission.

Vaara et al. [12] performed a prospective observational cohort study (the FINNAKI study) in 17 Finnish ICUs from September 2011 to February 2012. These authors analyzed data from 283 critically ill patients with AKI (without preexisting CKD) requiring RRT, 26.9 % of which had fluid overload at the initiation of RRT, were admitted more often for sepsis (25.0 % vs. 8.2 %, $p<0.001$), and had a higher hospital mortality (56.6 % vs. 23.7 %, $p<0.001$).

Silversides et al. [13] analyzed data from 492 critically ill patients with AKI. The median daily fluid balance was significantly different between patients who died in hospital (1,134 mL, interquartile range [IQR] 242–2,556 mL) and survivors (413 mL, IQR −371 to 1,106 mL) ($p<0.01$). A positive fluid balance was an independent risk factor for mortality (adjusted OR per 1,000 mL more positive fluid balance 1.36, 95 % CI 1.18–1.57, $p=0.001$).

These results were pooled together in a recent meta-analysis that included 12 cohort studies [14]. Data on mortality were reported by six studies, and fluid overload was significantly associated with an increased risk of death (cumulative OR 2.23, 95 % CI 1.66–3.01).

However, it is not clear whether fluid overload is a cause of increased mortality or rather a marker of illness severity, or both. Only RCTs can address this issue.

22.3.2.2 High-Volume Hydration in Patients Undergoing Percutaneous Coronary Intervention

As mentioned above, CIN is a major concern in interventional cardiology. Patients suffering from acute myocardial infarction undergoing primary PCI have been shown to be at greater risk of developing AKI. The only recommended prevention regimen is moderate hydration. Manari at al. [15] conducted a multicenter RCT of 592 patients undergoing primary angioplasty in five Italian hospitals. Patients were assigned in a 1:1:1:1 ratio to: (a) normal saline 1 mL kg^{-1} h^{-1} for 12 h, (b) normal saline 3 mL kg^{-1} h^{-1} for 1 h and then 1 mL kg^{-1} h^{-1} for 11 h, (c) sodium bicarbonate solution 1 mL kg^{-1} h^{-1} for 12 h, (d) and sodium bicarbonate solution 3 mL kg^{-1} h^{-1} for 1 h and then 1 mL kg^{-1} h^{-1} for 11 h. Contrast-induced AKI developed in 18.1 % of patients, without statistically significant differences among treatment groups. Global 30-day and 1-year mortality were 2.8 % and 4.3 %, respectively, without any significant difference among groups. When groups were considered clustered together per hydration volume (normal [a+c] vs. high [b+d]), 30-day mortality was significantly higher in the high-volume hydration group ($p=0.04$), while only a trend toward increased 1-year mortality was found ($p=0.06$).

22.3.2.3 Prophylactic Sodium Bicarbonate in Cardiac Surgery

Sodium bicarbonate alkalinizes urine and slows down the Haber-Weiss reaction that generates reactive oxygen species via iron-dependent pathways. Moreover, it may also directly scavenge other reactive species from blood. Therefore, its administration might be beneficial to prevent AKI in those clinical situations in which iron-related oxidative stress may play a role in its development (i.e., cardiac surgery and CIN). Literature on this topic led to mixed results. Haase et al. [16] conducted a multicenter double-blinded RCT to investigate whether prophylactic administration of sodium bicarbonate in cardiac surgery can reduce the incidence of postoperative AKI. Three hundred fifty patients were randomized to receive either sodium bicarbonate or normal saline just after anesthesia induction and for the next 24 h. A total volume of 1.25 L was given to each patient, and a total dose of 5.1 mmol/kg sodium bicarbonate was administered to the treatment group. The study was stopped early under recommendation of the Data Safety and Monitoring Committee because interim analysis suggested likely lack of efficacy and possible harm. Although intention-to-treat analysis found that a greater proportion of patients in the bicarbonate group developed AKI (47.7 % vs. 36.4 %; OR 1.60, 95 % CI 1.04–2.45, $p=0.032$), the difference became nonsignificant after multivariable adjustment for group imbalances at baseline (OR 1.45, 95 % CI 0.90–2.33, $p=0.12$). In-hospital mortality was 6.3 % (11 patients) in the bicarbonate group and 1.7 % (3 patients) in the control group (OR 3.89, 95 % CI 1.07–14.20, $p=0.031$), while a not statistically significant difference in mortality was found at a longer follow-up (90-day mortality 7.5 % vs. 2.8 %; OR 2.76, 95 % CI 0.96–7.92, $p=0.056$).

Conclusion

Since the first international web-based Consensus Conference on mortality reduction in patients with or at risk for AKI was held, 13 more papers, dealing with ten interventions, have been published in a peer-reviewed journal showing a statistical significant effect on survival in patients with or at risk for AKI. Seven interventions might increase survival: preoperative RAS-I and aspirin, aprotinin, and sedation with dexmedetomidine in cardiac surgery, CRRT before and after PCI, ACEI in patients with AKI needing RRT, and HVHF in SAP. Three interventions might increase mortality: fluid overload in AKI patients, high-volume hydration before PCI, and prophylactic sodium bicarbonate in cardiac surgery. However, the overall quality of these studies is low. Only two interventions (CRRT before PCI and fluid overload) were already included in the Consensus Conference, and their possible role in affecting mortality of AKI patients is to some extent strengthened by the new studies identified. The others represent new hints for future research.

References

1. Landoni G, Bove T, Székely A et al (2013) Reducing mortality in acute kidney injury patients: systematic review and international web-based survey. J Cardiothorac Vasc Anesth 27:1384–1398
2. Bellomo R, Weinberg L (2012) Web-enabled democracy-based consensus in perioperative medicine: sedation or solution? J Cardiothorac Vasc Anesth 26:762–763
3. Greco M, Zangrillo A, Mucchetti M et al (2015) Democracy-based consensus in medicine. J Cardiothorac Vasc Anesth 29:506–509
4. Shi P, Li Z, Young N et al (2013) The effect of preoperative renin-angiotensin system inhibitors on outcomes in patients undergoing cardiac surgery. J Cardiothorac Vasc Anesth 27:703–709
5. Yao L, Young N, Liu H et al (2015) Evidence for preoperative aspirin improving major outcomes in patients with chronic kidney disease undergoing cardiac surgery: a cohort study. Ann Surg 261:207–212
6. Walkden GJ, Verheyden V, Goudie R et al (2013) Increased perioperative mortality following aprotinin withdrawal: a real-world analysis of blood management strategies in adult cardiac surgery. Intensive Care Med 39:1808–1817
7. Ji F, Li Z, Young N et al (2013) Post-bypass dexmedetomidine use and postoperative acute kidney injury in patients undergoing cardiac surgery with cardiopulmonary bypass. PLoS ONE 8:e77446
8. Spini V, Cecchi E, Chiostri M et al (2013) Effects of two different treatments with continuous renal replacement therapy in patients with chronic renal dysfunction submitted to coronary invasive procedures. J Invasive Cardiol 25:80–84
9. Wang AI, Bellomo R, Ninomiya T et al (2014) Angiotensin-converting enzyme inhibitor usage and acute kidney injury: a secondary analysis of RENAL study outcomes. Nephrology 19:617–622

10. Guo J, Huang W, Yang XN et al (2014) Short-term continuous high-volume hemofiltration on clinical outcomes of severe acute pancreatitis. Pancreas 43:250–254
11. Bellomo R, Cass A, Cole L et al (2012) An observational study fluid balance and patients outcomes in the randomized evaluation of normal vs. augmented level of replacement therapy trial. Crit Care Med 40:1753–1760
12. Vaara ST, Korhonen AM, Kaukonen KM et al (2012) Fluid overload is associated with an increased risk for 90-day mortality in critically ill patients with renal replacement therapy: data from the prospective FINNAKI study. Crit Care 16:R197
13. Silversides JA, Pinto R, Kuint R et al (2014) Fluid balance, intradialytic hypotension, and outcomes in critically ill patients with renal replacement therapy. Crit Care 18:624
14. Zhang L, Chen Z, Diao Y et al (2015) Association of fluid overload with mortality and kidney recovery in patients with acute kidney injury: a systematic review and meta-analysis. J Crit Care 30:860e7–860e13
15. Manari A, Magnavacchi P, Puggioni E et al (2014) Acute kidney injury after primary angioplasty: effect of different hydration treatments. J Cardiovasc Med 15:60–67
16. Haase M, Haase-Fielitz A, Plass M et al (2013) Prophylactic perioperative sodium bicarbonate to prevent acute kidney injury following open heart surgery: a multicenter double-blinded randomized controlled trial. PLoS Med 10:e1001426
17. Garg AX, Kurz A, Sessler DI et al (2014) Perioperative aspirin and clonidine and risk of acute kidney injury: a randomized clinical trial. JAMA 12:2254–2264
18. Fergusson DA, Hébert PC, Mazer CD et al (2008) A comparison of aprotinin and lysine analogues in high-risk cardiac surgery. N Engl J Med 29(358):2319–2331
19. The RENAL Replacement Therapy Study Investigators (2009) Intensity of continuous renal replacement therapy in critically ill patients. N Engl J Med 361:1627–1638

Index

© Springer International Publishing Switzerland 2016

G. Landoni et al. (eds.), *Reducing Mortality in Acute Kidney Injury*,
DOI 10.1007/978-3-319-33429-5

MIX
Papier aus verantwortungsvollen Quellen
Paper from responsible sources
FSC® C105338

If you have any concerns about our products,
you can contact us on
ProductSafety@springernature.com

In case Publisher is established outside the EU,
the EU authorized representative is:
Springer Nature Customer Service Center GmbH
Europaplatz 3, 69115 Heidelberg, Germany

Printed by Libri Plureos GmbH
in Hamburg, Germany